CHILDREN IN
THE HOSPITAL

CHILDREN IN THE HOSPITAL

by

Thesi Bergmann

in collaboration with

Anna Freud

INTERNATIONAL UNIVERSITIES PRESS, INC.
New York

Copyright 1965, by International Universities Press, Inc.

Library of Congress Catalog Card Number 65-28803

Manufactured in the United States of America
by Hallmark Press, New York

Contents

Foreword by ANNA FREUD	9
Foreword by THESI BERGMANN	11

Part I
The Hospital

1.	THE SETTING AT RAINBOW HOSPITAL	17
2.	RAINBOW AS A LONG-STAY HOSPITAL	19
3.	VISITING RULES	22
4.	ADMISSION PROCEDURES AND REACTIONS	26
5.	RELATIONS WITH THE NURSING STAFF	31
6.	RELATIONS WITH THE MEDICAL STAFF	35

Part II
The Child Patients

7.	PREPARATION FOR SURGERY	43
	Preparation and the Child's Age	46
	Some Examples of Preparation	48
	An Example of Successful Preparation	48
	A Successful Preparation at Slow Pace	51
	Unsuccessful Preparation of a Three-year-old	53
	Despair Not Lessened by Preparation	54
	Preparation by Reality Confrontation	55
	Necessary Preparations for Minor Events	57
8.	TYPICAL REACTIONS TO SPECIFIC ILLNESSES	59
	Orthopedic Patients	59
	Acceptance Based on Fantasy	61

	Breakdown of Acceptance	62
	Revolt during Recovery	64
	Reactions to Removal of Cast	65
	Other Effects of Motor Restraint	67
	Cardiac Patients	68
9.	SOME REACTIONS TO OTHER AFFLICTIONS	72
	The Impact of Blindness	73
	The Impact of Amputation	74
	The Impact of Death	76
10.	ILLNESS MISUNDERSTOOD AS PUNISHMENT	80
11.	DENIALS, REGRESSIONS, OTHER DEFENSIVE DEVICES, AND CONSTRUCTIVE RESOURCES	89
	Denial and Nightmares	90
	Denial by Fantasy	93
	Withdrawal and Reversal	93
	Adaptation by Regression	94
	An Example of Mastery	95
12.	ILLNESS AND PERSONALITY DEVELOPMENT	100
	Physical Illness as a Destructive Force	101
	Triumph of the Mind over Illness	106
	An Institutionalized Ill Child	111
13.	ARTHRITIC AND ASTHMATIC PATIENTS: INVOLVEMENT WITH THE MOTHER	117
	Arthritic Children	117
	Asthmatic Children	122
14.	RETURN HOME	129

Part III
Conclusion

15.	CONCLUSION	135
	Severe, Chronic versus Minor, Acute Illness	135
	Interaction between Mind and Body	141
	The Technique of "Mental First Aid" in the Children's Hospital	145
	A Future Technique of "Mental First Aid"	150
	LIST OF CASE ILLUSTRATIONS	153
	INDEX	156

Foreword

By now, the insights contained in psychoanalytic child psychology have been used for the handling of children in many areas, for their upbringing in home and school, their management in health and sickness, for child law and adoptive procedures. The opening up of every additional field always has been due to the efforts of some interested individual who applied himself to it singlehandedly, devotedly, and without much recognition until others followed suit. This, exactly, is the manner in which Thesi Bergmann took up work with chronically ill children, to pursue it quietly and unobtrusively, over almost twenty years, collecting data concerning their behavior, increasing understanding of their plight, and helping them to improve their fate.

It is my respect and appreciation for labors of this kind which have prompted me to join forces with her in shaping her findings for publication. While the material in this book and many of the conclusions drawn from it are wholly hers, the formulation of the text, the responsibility for the final selection from her examples, and the concluding chapter are wholly mine. I have done this work in the hope that the reader will enjoy the excellence of her observations, follow her argumentation, and profit in his own work from her experiences.

ANNA FREUD, LL.D., Sc.D.

Baltimore, County Cork, April, 1965

Foreword

The experiences of which I give account in the following pages have been collected during a period of almost twenty years, mainly at Rainbow Hospital which is one of the University Hospitals of Cleveland, Ohio. I owe gratitude to the physicians and nurses of that hospital as well as to the children and parents with whom I came in contact and who made my observations possible. As these records stand, they represent informal attempts to illustrate the everyday experiences of hospitalized children, their reactions to long-lasting illness, to medical treatment and surgical intervention, to discomfort and deprivation, as well as their adjustment to separation from home and to experiences of a new and unaccustomed kind. For my understanding of the children's attitude and behavior, I drew on the psychoanalytic theory of child development for which work of this kind opens up a new and promising field of application.

Although I was employed by the hospital authorities as a child therapist, this title is a misleading one. Neither the circumstances nor the nature of my task could, in fact, be summed up under this category. Child therapy is the term known to cover the various methods used to treat mental disturbance in childhood, whether this consists of deviations from the norm in growth and development, of arrests or disturbances of adaptation, pathological character formation or symptomatology. Its aim is the restoring of normal development, its duration is determined by the type or the severity of illness. It is obvious that none of these definitions fit my interactions with the young patients, which were more in the nature of offering first aid in the emergencies created by traumatic situations.

There were many children whose behavior was dominated by anxiety and for whom reassurance and guidance based on understanding were the appropriate means of facilitating adaptation. There were others whose latent conflicts had become activated and heightened by illness, hospitalization, and immobilization to a degree which threatened the success of hospital treatment and obstructed the child's path to recovery; with them, alleviation of the immediate difficulty became the imperative concern. In both instances watching the child patient's behavior, listening to his complaints, and, above all, establishing contact with him served as the source of information. In making such contact it helped that in my particular role I was not involved with physical manipulations or with any of the demands and restrictions placed on the child by the specific nature of his illness.

I found that, apart from helping the children, a "hospital therapist" is also in the position to assist parents, physicians, and nurses in their various roles.

Parents, especially mothers, were of course first and foremost concerned with their children's physical condition which had aroused their alarm and about which they required information, explanations, and, at times, reassurance. But, after danger had been overcome, or anxiety lessened, many also welcomed the opportunity to clarify other matters concerning their children, i.e., matters which were unrelated to the physical illness and had given cause for anxiety. What I had learned about the individual child in the hospital while following him through physical treatment, recovery, and convalescence thus became useful to the parent in understanding developmental problems, upsets, conflicts, difficulties in the parent-child relationship. Where the hospital experience revealed deep-seated abnormalities of the child, it was occasionally possible to introduce the idea of future therapy, i.e., to prepare the parents as well as the patient himself for entry into child analysis at a later date.

Similarly, information about the child, collected by me, could be passed on to those physicians who were aware of the patient's emotional reactions and their impact on adjustment to therapy and on recovery. Since the nature of the physician's or surgeon's own role often precludes intimacy with the patient, the therapist's role as a link in the doctor-patient relationship is an important one.

It was no less rewarding to share information with the nursing personnel whose task of enforcing the medical demands on the child was made easier where the patients' obstructive behavior, their noncooperation, their dependencies, their incessant demands could be explained and understood as the result of typical developmental attitudes and conflicts, as manifest reflections of latent complexes, as results of previous experiences, etc. While what I had to offer could often be used to advantage by the nurses in their handling of the patients, in return the observations made by the nursing personnel often made important and valuable contributions to my own work.

For the hospital therapist it is important to remember the limits which the conditions of the work automatically impose on her endeavor. Foremost among these is the fact that contact ceases when the set goal of physical improvement is reached and the patient leaves the hospital, whatever his emotional needs may be at that moment. What I was not permitted to forget was the fact that *emotional first aid* in the hospital is an adjunct to the total hospital experience and not an aim or a method which exists independently and in its own right.

THESI BERGMANN

Cleveland, April, 1965

Part I
THE HOSPITAL

1

The Setting at Rainbow Hospital

Rainbow Hospital is situated in South Euclid, a suburb of Cleveland, amid lawns, shrubs, and woods which convey a country atmosphere and are a welcome change for children transferred from city hospitals. While patients are still confined to their beds, they begin to anticipate playing outdoors; when this actually happens, they understand it as an important step in their recovery.

The hospital can accommodate approximately fifty patients—babies and children up to the age of sixteen. Most of them receive treatment or are in convalescence for corrective surgery for such diseases as poliomyelitis, Guillain-Barré syndrome, congenital malformations, tuberculosis of the bones and joints, Legg-Perthes disease, muscular dystrophy, rheumatoid arthritis, and various kinds of heart disease.

During my period of work, the majority of children

came, not directly from home, but from Babies' and Children's Hospital (B. & C. of University Hospitals) or from other affiliated hospitals where diagnostic examinations had been made, surgery performed, and the most acute phase of the illness treated. Referral took place at a point when the children were ready to participate in a more active regime and when, except in arthritic conditions and asthma, severe pains had ceased. According to age, the patients were distributed among five wards: the Nursery Ward (both sexes), Younger Boys' Ward, Older Boys' Ward, Younger Girls' Ward, Older Girls' Ward. (Although the bigger boys and girls also enjoyed each other's company during activities, separation of the sexes seemed to be welcomed at other times.)

Children under orthopedic care were immobilized in plaster casts for long first phases of treatment, recovery of functions taking place gradually in a second phase through exercise and pool activity. Children who had had acute heart disease observed a similar routine, complete bed rest being followed by gradual return to normal activity. For the whole period of convalescence they remained under the same physician who had attended them in the acute phase. When repetition of surgery became necessary, the patients returned to their hospitals of referral, as did patients who suffered a relapse after discharge from Rainbow. If necessary, they were then readmitted to Rainbow, readmission taking place sometimes after an interval of several years.

2

Rainbow as a Long-Stay Hospital

Although some children remained for a few weeks only (to complete convalescence or to await evaluation for further rehabilitation), the majority stayed for months (in plaster after corrective surgery) or even years (Legg-Perthes disease, tuberculosis). Accordingly, Rainbow had to take on the functions of a long-stay hospital, i.e., to provide not only for physical recovery but also for the mental growth and upbringing of its patients, the latter tasks being subsidiary to but no less important than the former one.

Since, traditionally, a child's need for tuition receives attention first, the local Board of Education had cooperated in establishing and supervising hospital schooling, graded from nursery school upward to junior high. Two hours of daily instruction in small groups, with a great deal of individual attention, enabled most children to keep pace with their age groups.

It proved less easy, and more revolutionary, to provide also for the children's emotional and personality growth, neither of which is at a standstill during illness but for which the hospital setting, even at its best, cannot offer normal or wholly suitable conditions. Hospital life is artificial and overprotective when compared with home life. The importance of the ill body and its needs takes precedence, of necessity, over the mental needs, medical prescription and nursing routine assuming the place of importance usually held by convention and morality. The authority of doctors and nurses supersedes that of the parents. Group life replaces the intimacy of the mother-child or family relationship, the community setting being very acceptable to some older age groups and wholly unsuitable for the younger ones. Identifications are made with the roles and activities of the staff rather than with their personal qualities. In short, while the children pass through the same phases of drive and emotional development which they would pass through at home, growth appears distorted in two directions, once through the mere fact of physical disability, secondly by the inevitable environmental alterations.

Under such circumstances, efforts of the entire hospital personnel were needed to restore and maintain normality. In Rainbow, physicians, nurses, and therapist combined forces in their attempts to mold an institution into the semblance of a home and to provide programs and conditions which coincided, at least approximately, with the established needs of child development. That the atmosphere in Rainbow is peaceful and unhurried, compared with that of most large general hospitals, may have been a considerable asset in this respect.

3

Visiting Rules

Psychoanalytic child psychology leaves no doubt that children are emotionally dependent on their parents and that this dependence is necessary for purposes of normal development; also, that relationships in a hospital are, at best, poor substitutes for family relationships. Once these facts are accepted, relaxation of visiting rules becomes an inevitable consequence.

In Rainbow, parents were given every opportunity to visit their children any time they liked, and to observe them during stressful as well as during easy times, in periods of physical therapy, pool activity, exercises, school, play, etc. Care was taken that parents and children could interact as they do at home, a child occasionally preferring to play with other children while the mother visited with other mothers or the nurse. Young children were especially eager to be put to bed and tucked in by their mothers, while older children preferred to be up with their visitors as long as possible. When there were no epidemics in the community, siblings visited on Sunday, which often became "picnic day" for the whole family in the hospital grounds.

Family ties were maintained further by the children making telephone calls to their homes and by all, except those in body casts, if they had progressed sufficiently in convalescence, going home occasionally for week ends. The latter visits were effective in teaching the child to cope with his disabilities under the less protective circumstances of a normal home, to mix with friends and neighbors after a prolonged absence, to be seen by them in a wheel chair, walking with braces or crutches, etc. Parents became accustomed in this manner to deal on their own with the responsibility of caring for a frail or handicapped child and to master their own anxieties.

Links between hospital and home regimes were also forged by including the visiting mothers in observing and discussing the children's many idiosyncrasies, especially the numerous food fads and eating difficulties which occur in many normal children but which are particularly numerous in and significant for the ill child. What the hospital demonstrated in this respect was how to avoid crying and tearful scenes at mealtimes; how to encourage appetite while eliminating all pressure, by respecting and following the child's expressed likes and dislikes, by introducing self-selection, servings in minute quantity, etc. Although initially surprised and doubtful, mothers usually did not find it too difficult to adopt similar ways of handling eating problems at home.

While the nurses were better equipped than the mothers to approach some difficulties, especially those in the area of infantile eating disturbances, there were other problems and difficult situations which the nursing staff could not solve adequately without having recourse to the mother's help and her own immediate contact with the child, as the following example shows:

SHIRLEY, five years old, was admitted to Rainbow with Legg-Perthes disease, of which she herself was oblivious since she suffered neither pain nor discomfort from it. Accordingly, she could not understand and was in revolt against her leg being kept in traction, off the ground, etc. Whenever she found herself unobserved, she got out of bed and, when reproached, reiterated indignantly: "But I *can* walk—I walk since I was a little baby." Finally, in desperation, the nurses put a small restraining vest on her, with ribbons tied to the bed, a measure which Shirley hated and understood as punishment.

The situation became worse when the mother obviously shared the child's feeling, relieved her of the garment which she called "disgraceful," and threatened to cease visiting unless the vest was removed and the child became good, i.e., immobile, a promise which Shirley made but was unable to keep.

What was needed in this impasse between mother, child, and hospital was my intervention in three directions. While the nurses were asked to suspend action, Shirley was shown how much she wanted her mother to protect her against the "meanness" of the hospital staff. The mother, on the other hand, was shown the necessity to keep her child off her feet to effect a cure, and that only her own wholehearted acceptance of this restriction could make the child conform. She admitted that she herself had felt humiliated by the appearance of the vest and included in Shirley's "punishment" for not having brought up a more compliant child. When the mother was reassured that none of this was her fault and that Shirley's revolt was age adequate for a high-spirited, independent five-year-old, she became able to handle the situation; i.e., she herself refastened the vest on the child, explaining gently that this was no punishment but an aid to quicker recovery, how much she wanted Shirley to be well and strong, how hard it must be for her to stay in bed, etc. Miraculously enough, with the mother's acceptance, Shirley became able to comply.

4

Admission Procedures and Reactions

In keeping with the general atmosphere at Rainbow, admission procedures were informal and deliberately leisurely. Instead of being asked questions, child and parent were taken around the premises and the new situation presented to them in concrete and, so far as possible, favorable terms. While the physical therapy department and the bathing pool aroused the curiosity of all children, the older ones especially were reassured by the familiar sight of a schoolroom and by the news that there would be weekly movies, meetings of Brownies, Cubs, and Scouts, frequent visiting, etc. While serving the purpose of reassurance for the newcomer, this "tour" of the hospital also provided information to the staff concerning his habits, predilections, and dislikes, his suitability for being placed with one or the other group or neighbor, his reaction to his illness, indications of the support needed, etc.

This form of introduction usually carried out by the head nurse, was appreciated by children and parents alike as instrumental in lessening the fear of parting. Mothers would say: "She is a good nurse, she talks to you" or "She must be a mother herself, she knows how one feels."

In spite of all the precautions taken when the patient entered Rainbow, we were not allowed to forget that we were not the first hospital with which the child had had contact and that earlier admissions had taken place in very different circumstances. Many of our children had been rushed to the hospital in the first instance in emergencies, very ill, in great pain. They had sensed the distress of their parents, watched their fear, excitement, sense of urgency while hospitalization was arranged, and added these to their own bewilderment and separation terror. Where no emergency had existed, the older children had derived some comfort from previous explanations and from their understanding of necessary procedures; but even for these children the unfamiliar sights, sounds, and experiences with which they were confronted seldom coincided with what they had anticipated. The younger ones gave every sign of having been helplessly exposed to overpowering anxieties, increased by strange beds, strange foods, and strangers' faces.

Children do not react with increased familiarity when exposed to repeated surgery or transferred to a second hospital. On the contrary, sensitized by their initial experience, it is common for them to meet every subsequent operation with increased anxiety or to enter any subsequent hospital with increased resentment. Notwithstanding the fact that at this juncture the illness may be less acute, fears and anxieties belonging to the former occasion are revived. Besides, change of routine is experienced as disturbing, familiar figures of doctors, nurses, and fellow patients are missed, and hopes for an early return home are shattered. However pleasant the new hospital surroundings, what they offer the patient seems above all a prolonged term of imprisonment.

Understanding the children's attitude in this respect, we learned at Rainbow to meet and react to various types of behavior in newcomers. Some children expressed anxiety and resentment openly, cried, screamed, refused treatment as well as consolation. They watched their fellow patients as if terrorized, expecting that all the painful procedures they saw would also be applied to them. This created difficulties in the ward where they upset the other patients. We recognized it as necessary to arrange for privacy where the upset could be allowed to run its course in the comforting presence of either parent, nurse, or therapist. Surprisingly enough, in time, these same children became the most accepting of medical care and the limitations imposed on them, as if the unrestrained discharge of fear, despair, and rage had also left them free to cope with the situation by more positive means.

A striking contrast to these initial reactions of extreme upset was offered by the so-called "perfect" patients. These were children who appeared to submit to the experience with calm resignation; their behavior was cheerful, understanding, and cooperative; they were dominated by the wish to get well and mustered all necessary resources under the impact of this wish. Only later did we discover that these children did not dare to face up to the overwhelming feelings evoked by their situation and that they used all their available energy to defend themselves against danger, anxieties, and frightening fantasies. Such defenses broke down promptly as soon as the immediate danger was removed, and the denied emotional content returned with a vengeance, incapacitating the patient.

It was predominantly with this latter type of child that various quasi-pathological reactions could be observed, such as regression to infantile modes of behavior, wetting and soiling, eating or sleeping difficulties, learning inhibitions. Restriction of motility, a part of many treatment procedures, left no active outlet for pent-up emotions and aggressions and enforced the child's resorting to temper tantrums and abusive language.

We also learned to dread, as especially endangered, the depressed children who felt abandoned and, instead of revolting, resigned themselves to their fate. They presented no difficulty for the hospital routine since they were quiet, obedient, and submissive, to the extent that their plight was often overlooked. Their specific reaction was that of emotional withdrawal; i.e., they were loosening their ties with their legitimate love objects and concentrating their feelings on their own selves, or on their bodies, or on their fantasies. Although the harmful effect of this might remain hidden while they were in the hospital, it became obvious after their return home, when such children showed aftereffects in their relationships, sometimes of frightening proportion and of long duration.

In Rainbow, as in other long-stay hospitals, we also had the opportunity to watch the children cope with and overcome their initial emotional upset and to settle down in the hospital atmosphere in spite of the initial turmoil caused by illness, anxiety, separation from home, and adjustment to strange people. It speaks for the normal child's versatility and adaptability that even severely upsetting experiences can be weathered provided that an adequate measure of support, understanding, and comfort is forthcoming from the environment.

5

Relations with the Nursing Staff

From school age onward, children become accustomed to intermittent absences from home, at least in the daytime. They also acquire, in addition to the distinction between the mother's and the father's roles, a growing awareness of the specialized functions which different adults can fulfill for them. Normally, a child does not expect the same from father and mother, does not expect from the teacher what the parent does for him, or vice versa. This prepares him, at least so far as understanding goes, for accepting the nurse as being knowledgeable about body ailments and able to give relief in situations of physical distress which go beyond the parents' ability to help. Once the children had realized the nurse's superior competence and experienced her ability to give as much body comfort as circumstances permitted, we found that the older ones became willing to accept her as the adult in authority, who was responsible for carrying out doctor's orders, whose ruling had to be submitted to in matters of body care. This point was reached all the quicker, the more obviously the parents trusted the nursing arrangements made in behalf of the child. Where such trust was absent and loyalty conflicts intervened, the patients were apt to behave more obstructively, more disobediently, etc.

In complete contrast to these comparatively straightforward situations, an effective all-round nursing of the youngest children presented an almost superhuman task. A toddler, whose body has been completely in his mother's care, is unable to understand why this care should be relinquished by her just at the point when his need for it is greatest, why his distress needs to be increased by unfamiliar handling. No child under the ages of three or four can therefore be expected to react positively to a nurse's intervention and to cooperate with her. For the nurse this creates the anomalous situation that, while complete devotion to a helpless patient is demanded of her, no affectionate or even remotely grateful return is made by a youngster who regards her with hostility, resents her presence as usurping his own mother's place, and rejects her efforts at giving comfort and consolation by persisting in unrelieved separation distress.

The nurses found it helpful when these difficulties were brought into the open and discussed with them; they began to understand that the difficulties were not due to the individual worker's shortcomings or incapacity but were inevitable occurrences based on fateful interference with the young child's overriding need for his mother's presence. In the severe illnesses we had to deal with, where the situation was fraught with danger to the child's life or whole future capability, many mothers were relieved to hand over responsibility; this did not alter the fact that their toddlers were unable to transfer their allegiance, their trust, their dependence, and their emotional ties at the same pace.

On the other hand, there were also cases, such as Ronnie's, where the nurse's understanding and capacity were acceptable to the child in the face of his own mother's helplessness, and where, consequently, a feeling of fulfillment and success accompanied the nursing even of the very young.

RONNIE was a boy of two and a half, who had been rushed to the hospital with acute poliomyelitis. Although his mother was permitted to remain with him, she had to leave him often to take care of her home and her other young children. Bewildered by illness and separation from home, Ronnie refused to eat and regressed so far as drinking from a cup was concerned, taking only small quantities of milk from a bottle. Since his toilet training had been strict and established early, he did not, like many other children, express his distress by wetting and soiling but ceased to void altogether. Since there was no physical basis for either of these reactions, we assumed that they represented a solution of his conflict, i.e., conflict between a powerful urge to regress to messing and an equally powerful fear of displeasing his orderly mother who—according to his imaginings—had already shown her displeasure with him by banishing him from home.

In this impasse a nurse took over. She was advised to disregard cleanliness and to allow him to handle and mess with food to the extent that he needed a complete cleanup after each attempted meal. The cheerful and unconcerned manner in which she dealt with his messiness obviously lessened his fear of wetting and enabled him after a while to use the bedpan. She showed equal permissiveness with regard to other regressions to infantile behavior such as clinging, being cared for passively, of which his mother would have disapproved strongly.

Under these conditions, Ronnie formed a strong attachment to the nurse and refused all help from the mother, beginning to cry immediately when she handled him. This distressed her, in turn, and she needed reassurance. It was explained that at this juncture her horror of his bad eating manners was out of place, that at this point the demand for both clean toilet and table habits would lead only to refusal of function, that babyish behavior would not be permanent, that attachment to the nurse was no more than a means to the end of regaining health, etc.

Actually, during the period of recovery, and under the nurse's guidance, Ronnie relearned to function adequately, according to his mother's training. He was able to pick up development at the point where illness had stopped him in his tracks. Once again he trustfully turned to his mother, while the nurse, according to plan, stepped out of his life.

6

Relations with the Medical Staff

In Rainbow, nurses and therapist had the great advantage of working with a medical staff interested not only in their specialized medical field but in the children's general welfare. They were knowledgeable about the far-reaching interactions between mind and body, the importance of the mother's and child's relationship to them, its impact on the patients' ability to cope with pain and submit to restrictions, and the innumerable detailed ways in which physical discomfort can be either alleviated or aggravated by a child's emotional position. They were equally aware of the fact that, however carefully and considerately they themselves approached and handled the children, the patients' attitude to them was determined in equal measure by whatever experience they had had with family doctors or pediatricians in their earlier lives before hospitalization.

The children with whom we dealt at Rainbow arrived with very different backgrounds in this respect. Some had been brought up from birth under the guidance of pediatrician and well-baby clinic whom the mother trusted, respected, and accepted as benevolent authorities in health as well as in illness, an attitude which was carried over to the hospital and usually persisted throughout the most stressful and critical periods of the child's illness. For these children, the physician was usually an object of admiration and for identification, sometimes a figure of awe, respected for his knowledge of the body and its functioning, envied for his possession of desirable instruments, and often endowed with omnipotence, i.e., the magical power to "make people well."

In contrast, there also were children in whose lives medical visits had been rare occurrences, experienced by parents and child as a necessary evil. Such mothers usually feared being blamed by the medical authorities for some negligence or general lack of care; their children often felt guilty for having caused damage to their own bodies (by masturbation, by other real or imaginary acts of disobedience) and expected to be found out and punished when examined. These children also carried their former attitudes into the hospital, to the detriment of their relations with the medical staff, toward whom they remained for long periods aloof or hostile, frightened or distrustful.

On the other hand, we would have erred in the hospital if we had regarded all the attitudes the children displayed to their doctors as derived from past experiences, or from identification with their parents, or even from the child's rational understanding of the physicians' or surgeons' role in physical reality. Much of their behavior had to be understood in the unrealistic terms of age-adequate emotions, drive components, complexes and conflicts such as the expression of fears of mutilation and amputation (the surgeon seen as the punishing castrator at the height of the boy's positive oedipus complex); as the expression of masochistic tendencies (in girls with strong passive components or boys in the negative oedipal phase); as a bid for admiration (for heroic endurance); for passive dependence on the doctor (who "owns" the child's body as a successor to or substitute for the parent), etc.

That painful experiences can arouse powerful masochistic tendencies in children, who then become passively tied to the originator of pain, discomfort, and deprivation, was illustrated by the case of DONNA, a girl of ten, afflicted with tuberculosis of the spine. She was devoted to her physician as shown by comments such as: "There is only one thing here that I like—I am only waiting for my doctor's visits—I love it when he comes to see me." Despite all the hardship he had to inflict on her in treatment, several operations included, her entire interest was centered around him, and her anxieties around his decisions were mingled with pleasure. Far from dreading him, she expressed only deep and genuine gratitude for "her doctor."[1]

GEORGE, a boy of eight, suffering from the effects of Guillain-Barré, also looked forward to his doctor's visits, but the reasons for his cheerful anticipation were different from Donna's. Although these visits were accompanied by

[1] For further observations of Donna, see Chapters 8 and 11.

minor but painful procedures, he did not appear to mind. "Hi! Where is he? It's Wednesday. Why is he not here?" Obviously, he was willing to accept some anxious anticipation for the sake of the opportunity to show off his manliness and powers of endurance in front of an admired and respected person.

Some children also enjoyed their doctor's concern in the same manner as, at home, they enjoyed their parents' solicitude. Others, who had been neglected and deprived at home, became almost elated at the sudden realization that here were people who were devoted to their welfare, and they responded to such interest with loyalty toward the medical staff and devotion on their part.

Nevertheless, after repeated hospitalizations, some children also became aware of the painful fact that such enjoyable contacts did not last and that it might be less painful in the long run to ward off relations from the outset than to have them broken off after they had been formed.

An example of this negativistic attitude was given by EVE, aged twelve. She had had many recurrences of severe heart disease. During doctors' visits she pretended not to pay any attention to their presence and to be engrossed in reading. Afterward she would mimic their conversation: "Says the little boss, 'She is doing fine.' Says the big boss, 'Splendid, would you like some more uptime?' Says the little boss, 'Half an hour?' What do they know? Half an hour! Who cares? Would I like that? I am going to stay in my bed—just because."

Commonly, the doctor-patient relationships underwent a radical change with the beginning of convalescence proper when medication and treatment were decreased, uptime and activities increased, week ends at home arranged, and the time for discharge drew nearer. At this time older children liked to discuss the condition of their illness with their doctor, showed interest in their X-rays, past and future progress, further regimes, etc. Once anxieties had subsided, realistic appraisals of the situation could take their place. But at all times children could be seen intently watching the expression on their doctors' faces and listening to their conversations, in the hope of finding some clue to answer the eternal questions: "Am I all right? When can I go home?"

Part II
THE CHILD PATIENTS

7

Preparation for Surgery

In the not-too-distant past, children of all ages were taken to the operation room, unaware of what was going to happen to them. It was thought kinder, at that time, not to excite their fearful expectations beforehand, or even to discuss afterward the experience which, it was hoped, they would soon forget but which, on the contrary, often proved to be traumatic and to have lasting consequences.

More recently, it has been established as every child's right to be prepared for the event, the duty to do so being shared equally by parents, doctors, and hospital staff. Such preparations are not easy, even when they concern such minor interventions as removal of tonsils or adenoids, repair of hernias, etc. They become formidable tasks in the severe conditions with which we had to deal, where the outcome of an operation is often unpredictable and nothing can be foreseen as certain except acute pain and ordeals of long duration. It is difficult for the worker under such circumstances to combine honesty with the necessary reassurance.

Any surgical intervention announced beforehand to adult or child arouses the patient's legitimate and conscious anticipation of pain, discomfort, deprivation, and often mutilation. While this is difficult for anybody to deal with, children, because of their more limited knowledge of the realities, are spared, perhaps, some of the agonizing appraisals of the situation. On the other hand, they are more easily overwhelmed by events since they are less tolerant of frustration, less equipped to cope with disasters, and their emotional balance, far from being stable, is overthrown by any increase of anxiety.

It is precisely in this respect that the child is at the greatest disadvantage. In his mind, where the dividing lines between conscious and unconscious, reality and fantasy, reason and affect, are less firmly established than they will be in later life, archaic fears and primitive anxieties from all levels of development merge only too readily with the real dangers and obscure the issue by confusing corrective surgery with punishment, operation with castration, and therapeutic procedures and manipulations with attack. It may be comparatively easy for a normal adult to be courageous in the face of surgery, i.e., to succeed in dealing with external threats in reality terms and on their own ground. The same attitude may be quite impossible for the child for whom these threats join forces with the many fantastic dangers lodged in the unconscious, where reason is ineffective and primitive reactions such as terror, panic, tantrums take over instead.

Ideally, to prepare adequately for surgery, the adult responsible should possess much information about the given child. He should know of external events such as surgery undergone by a relative or friend with whom the child, perhaps, identifies; its positive or negative result which may affect his expectation; previous information given to the child about the body and its functioning; previous surgery and the explanations and support given at that time. He should also know of internal facts such as the child's habitual resources and defenses in the face of danger; his developmental status with regard to drive and personality development, his dominant anxieties and fantasies. Only when a child's external and internal reality can be seen combined, in interaction with each other, is there a chance to predict approximately how he will translate happenings such as anesthesia, pain, physical damage, and immobilization into emotional experience.[1]

There are not many means by which parents, doctors, or hospital staff can combat the emotional upsets caused by this confusion between real and imaginary dangers. On the one hand, reality can be clarified by giving the child as complete and honest a picture of the forthcoming events as he can understand; this helps him enlist his own reason, insight, and good sense. On the other hand, the child can be steered toward a

[1] See Anna Freud: *Normality and Pathology in Childhood.* New York: International Universities Press, 1965.

frame of mind in which frightening fantasies—whatever their source and nature—are not denied but approached, faced, and verbalized. Even when no deliberate interpretation is given, this acts as reassurance, diminishes confusion and misunderstanding of facts, and decreases the power of distorting unconscious elements. Guided and supported in this manner, children are better able to hold their anxieties in check and to transform revolt or passive endurance into active cooperation.

As regards the length of time needed for such preparatory work with the child, it is by now common knowledge that individual children differ widely in this respect. While some profit from a slow approach and have to be led toward the thought of operation by minute steps, little by little, the given period being used to strengthen their resources, others become completely swamped by fears if handled in the same manner; for them, the preparation time has to be kept short to avoid the development of an unfortunate and unprofitable state of mind.

PREPARATION AND THE CHILD'S AGE

The preparation described is possible only with older children, of course, i.e., with those ages where verbal communication has been established and where reason is developing. There is no parallel method which can be used in the preverbal stages.

An appropriate form of assistance in the case of infants is to guide the mother, i.e., to approach her with the same combination of explanation of facts, correction of misunderstandings, elucidation of fantasies, honesty, and reassurance. This, in turn, helps her to support the child and, where such support is unfailing (and the mother available), it can be remarkably successful in carrying an infant more or less unharmed through the operative and postoperative phases.

The most endangered age group, on the other hand, are the toddlers (approximately one to two and a half or three years), who have the worst of both worlds in every respect. They are no longer wholly supported and protected against experience by their mothers but are too young to grasp with their own reason what is happening to them; they can neither express feelings verbally nor comprehend explanations, nor accept or deal with difficulties except by panic or massive regression. Very little is accomplished by the attempts to prepare them for surgery by using anticipatory play; whatever expectations are aroused by this never match the subsequent realities. Nevertheless it would be wrong to conclude that for them efforts at preparation should be abandoned. On the contrary, attempts to do it more successfully should be redoubled and experiments tried in all directions. Since it is especially the postoperative situation which becomes traumatic (finding themselves in traction, immobilized in a plaster cast, with an amputated limb, etc.), it is essential to extend help in that period and to find means to enable the children to cope with and assimilate such experiences. It is also the children in this age group who need their mothers' presence urgently, since their situation becomes unbearable if separation, i.e., desertion by the mother, is added gratuitously to the other, inevitable, hardships.

SOME EXAMPLES OF PREPARATION

Obviously, in the actuality of hospital work, it is more often than not impossible to maintain "ideal" conditions, i.e., to know enough about the individual children, their past, their personalities, their predominant fantasies, or always to have sufficient time to prepare them. In some cases, the surgeon, suddenly and quite unexpectedly, decided that surgery was urgently indicated. In others, a bed became available suddenly in the hospital where the operation was to be performed. But in these instances, too, the most important aspects of the situation had to be dealt with, even though the actions taken were sometimes different from what had seemed appropriate.

What follows are some actual cases encountered in the hospital. The way in which they were dealt with may serve to illustrate one or the other aspect of the problems mentioned.

An Example of Successful Preparation

At the age of eight LINDA, a spastic diplegic, was told about her approaching operation. She seemed to understand that the purpose of the operation was to improve her physical condition. She was full of joyful anticipation and reiterated again and again: "I am so happy, I am go-

PREPARATION FOR SURGERY   49

ing to have an operation." I would have been more inclined to take this at its face value if Linda had not earlier betrayed a different state of mind in a story she dictated, in which she left no doubt about her guilt feelings:

WHAT LINDA DOES AT HOME

Once there was a little girl and her name was Linda and she was very bad. So one day she thought of something. She wanted to pet the dog and she did not like the dog at all. And here the dog bit her. So she ran into the house crying. And then Mom asked what was wrong and she said, "The dog bit me." And Mummy put something on it. And she went out again and then she ran back into the house because she wanted to ask Mummy something: "Could I go and pat the dog?" And Mummy said, "You better not." And Linda insisted that she wanted to pat the dog again. And when she went out she thought she better not pat the dog this time, but she went out to play on the front lawn. And she saw a snake. So she ran into the house and did not go outdoors again that day.

THE END

"See," said Linda, "that was at home, really and truly when I was home."

I tried, in conversation, to penetrate and shake her "happiness," with the result that she succeeded finally in asking me innumerable questions which she had previously suppressed as too upsetting. Foremost among these was her worry about ether, a worry which she could diminish only when permitted a whiff of it in the laboratory. She then found it "not as bad as I thought."

Although Linda was essentially a fearful little girl, apt to shy away from dangers and to deny them, such simple methods and talks sufficed to enlist her cooperation in the operation and to prevent her anxieties from blotting out the expectation of improvement. That, simultaneously, she became realistically curious and also accepted her own discomfort and the sense of loneliness implied in the experience is borne out by her own final description of the event in which fear, inquisitiveness, and the wish to cope vie with each other.

MY BIG ADVENTURE

When my doctor told me that I should have an operation, I was very curious because I never before had an operation. I was quite happy about it because I never had an operation before and I wanted to know what it would be like. I was very curious. I was really a little scared because I never had an operation before. I was scared because I never had ether before and I was afraid I might feel it. I did not mind to go to St. Luke's. I thought it would be something real nice until they would take me to the operating room. You asked why I was so happy about the operation, but I said that I know that I would be all right after the operation. In a way I was a little bit scared, because I never had an operation before and did not know what it would be like. And then they took me to the operating room and put me on the table and laid me on my side on the table and put a kind of sand bag on the side to keep me on the side. I thought, "Where's the ether, where's the ether?" I asked, "Where is the ether?"

And the nurse said, "We will have it pretty soon." And then they put a white stand by the operating table. Then the nurse gave me a white mask to hold, but I did not want to hold it, so the nurse held it and took a bottle off the stand and she opened a little cover and the ether went on the mask. I fell asleep. It smelled awful and I could taste the air of it. When I got dizzy and started to go to sleep, I let out a yell. I dreamed that I had an operation. I can't remember anything of the operation. And then when I woke up, I asked if I had a cast on, and the nurse said, "Yes." Then I asked where my father and mother were. She said that they went down for a cup of coffee and that they would be right back. And when they came my father opened up a box and he took out my Toni doll. And I played with her and told Mummy and Daddy that she was very nice. They stayed with me until after supper. And that is about the operation. When I saw my cast, I said, "Oh, oh, oh." And it burned like fire where I was operated on.

A Successful Preparation at Slow Pace

HARRIET, a girl of thirteen, suffering from poliomyelitis, found it difficult to disentangle herself from castration fears and fantasies which had haunted her since early childhood and which increased when surgery was suggested to her. Her upbringing had been an unhappy one, filled with threats, excessive demands, and much distress.

When her physician suggested a muscle transplant to improve the use of her hands, she became despondent and was reported to have cried the rest of the day. Apparently, she did not believe that the operation would be comparatively small and expected and feared a more extensive procedure (all the more so because she knew that she had a slight anomaly of her sex organs).

Although the nature of the surgery had been explained to her in detail, she asked questions concerning it as soon as she came to see me. To find out the truth, she seemed to test whether everybody would say the same:

"Why would my hand be better? What's wrong?"

"These muscles do not work together and Dr. T. would correct this so that you could bring your little finger and thumb together. This would make it easier for you to write, to hold a knife or fork, to manage your crutches and many other things."

"How will he do it?"

"He would make a little cut here and—"

"I am sick and tired of hearing about that little cut. That's what you say, but no one knows what all they are going to cut and I do not need it. I am all right and if I pray hard enough, the Lord will help me and I know he is helping me—see—"

In her excitement and fear, Harriet held out the hand considered for surgery and, with perfection, did what she had been unable to do so far: she used her fingers correctly, bringing thumb and little finger together. This miraculous improvement, in some way probably made possible by the tremendous emotional upheaval, lasted about three weeks, then dwindled away slowly, and left her very desolate and in need of comfort.

During the subsequent year any discussion of surgery was suspended, although she was given to understand that the surgeon was ready to operate whenever she wanted it. But in spite of many improvements (better walking on crutches, freer movement of the arms, a more pleasing personal appearance, etc.) the fear of the "cut" remained. Although she permitted the young hospital aides to advise her about clothes in the attempt to change her into a "glamor girl," she firmly resisted having her hair shortened and wore it instead in two straggly, untidy braids.

Finally, by openly discussing and clarifying her castration fear in her interviews with me, she became able to approach the situation realistically. She first agreed to have her hair trimmed evenly, then to have it cut shorter and shorter, and finally talked about the operation to improve the function of her hand. "Will you ask Dr. T. to do it?" she asked.

"He will be pleased if you ask him yourself."

In her case preparation for surgery had taken no less than a year.

Unsuccessful Preparation of a Three-year-old

JANE, a girl of three, was admitted to Rainbow for treatment of a congenital dislocated hip for which she had undergone many previous treatments, some of them apparently quite depriving and confining. Her initial stay with us was arranged to help prepare this frail child for her operation at Babies' and Children's Hospital, after which she was to return to us for prolonged convalescence.

While playing with her I tried to illustrate the various phases of surgery which she would experience. First, a little doll named Jane went in a car for a ride to another hospital. There the doll was put into a little bed and went to sleep. Jane put many plaster casts on the doll's "bad leg." Later we also put the doll on a frame and the leg in traction—all things that Jane herself would have to contend with. She proudly showed her doctor the little doll, took the plaster off many times during the day, and enjoyed applying a new cast. At the same time she herself was placed on a frame in order to acquaint her with this position. Although an hour would have been sufficient, she was apparently quite contented and wished to be left on it for a longer period.

According to the mother's reports, Jane did very well during her hospitalization at Babies' and Children's Hospital, where she stayed for less than a week. When she returned to Rainbow she asked for her doll, which like herself had her leg in plaster and also in traction; but although she looked at the doll with interest, she did not play. Instead, she worried us by becoming withdrawn, lying quietly on her frame for hours, looking at an old card or holding a toy brought by her mother. Although she would sing softly to herself, she showed no interest in anything else and merely sucked her thumb.

Obviously, in her case, preparation had proved ineffective, and the doll play, though pleasurable in itself, had failed to prepare her for the shock of immobilization during the postoperative phase.

Despair Not Lessened by Preparation

In the case of RUBY, aged four, preparation also proved ineffective when she was confronted with the results of surgery. Her leg was amputated for absent fibula at Babies' and Children's Hospital, where an extraordinarily kind and gentle resident had made efforts to prepare her for the event. After the operation she appeared to be content so long as her leg was invisible under the bandages; but whenever these had to be changed, she broke down and was inconsolable. On one of these occasions I held her on my lap and all I could do was to allow her deep despair to run its course. Finally, when she had calmed down a little, I attempted to help her toward verbal expression by asking: "What is it?" Trying to compose herself, she said, "Somebody took a scissors and cut my foot off." She seemed lost and forlorn, grieving like a child who has lost a beloved person. There is, to my mind, no adequate preparation for shocks and losses of this kind.

Preparation by Reality Confrontation

JACKIE, a boy of five, underwent a spinal operation, a type of surgery usually performed on older children. He himself had requested to have his back "fixed" and appeared pleased when his wish was granted so that he could be "like other little boys."

He came to Rainbow to see where he would live for some months after his operation, but this visit was arranged for him primarily so that he could meet children who were convalescing in body casts and become acquainted with the situation he himself would experience. These patients talked freely with Jackie, who seemed to be quite unafraid. The next day he was admitted to Babies' and Children's Hospital, where thoughtful explanations were given to him in preparation for surgery.

In one of our first meetings after he came to Rainbow for his convalescence he painted a picture—big blobs of all colors. When he announced that the picture was finished, I asked, "Well, and what is the story of your picture?"

"This is a map," he replied.

"Yes, it does look like a map. Is it to be used on a trip?"

"This is a map of my operation," he said, "and I want you to send it to Dr. B. so that he can show the map to little children when he tells them about the operation." He proceeded to dictate a letter to accompany the map:

> This is a map of my operation. They fixed a bone. And they put stitches in it. They put a bandage over the stitches. Then they took the stitches out and put a cast on me. The blue is what the bones they fixed. And the green is what they put the stitches on. The brown is the shots. I took some oxygen. They mixed the oxygen in a sort of space-mask and this is the color pink. Now I woke up and went to recovery. Dr. B. was in the recovery room and the nurse and I, and this is the color yellow. Now I took another medication that took my pain. I think that is about all.

With him, preparation which consisted entirely of the explanation of real facts served to produce a satisfactory acceptance of the postoperative situation.

Confrontation with other patients' experiences often proves helpful as a preparation, especially in cases of surgery of the spine, a fusion to correct scoliosis. The operation effects such striking changes in appearance that adolescents, allowed to watch the transformation in a fellow patient, become filled with happy anticipation. Girls compare the body cast with a "cocoon" from which the butterfly emerges as a completely different being. Such aspects of the situation lessen the fear of the heavy cast in which the child has to remain for almost six months.

Necessary Preparations for Minor Events

MARION, aged seven years, who suffered from very severe asthma, required different handling. While living at Rainbow she did not have the frightening attacks which were frequent occurrences at home. Because she received no treatment or medication for asthma and because she felt relatively well, she denied her knowledge of being in a hospital with other sick children and acted as though she were in a boarding school. I saw it as my task to help her face her real situation. Having undergone numerous tests and biopsies throughout her life and having been exposed to many frightening situations during previous hospitalizations when she had been desperately ill, she dreaded the mere finger prick involved in the taking of a blood sample, and was known at Babies' and Children's Hospital for becoming extremely disturbed and difficult on these occasions. I came to know her well enough to decide that I must prepare her as quickly as possible, so that she could not indulge in fantasies and become fearful.

I arranged to have the blood samples taken while I was present. When I picked her up from school, she remarked, "This is a nice school."

"I think you know, Marion, that this is really a hospital where children also go to school."

"You mean a hospital where they stick children with needles?"

"Yes, sometimes they have to have a sample of blood so that they know best how to make children get well again."

"Would they do it to me?"

"Yes."

"When?"

"Now."

"Where?"
"Here." (We had reached the laboratory.)
"I will scream."
"Yes, maybe it makes you feel better."

Marion sat down and held out her finger. She dutifully shouted, "Ouch," and said, "Is that all? I want to put the band aid on myself." A dreaded ordeal was over—Marion had not been promised anything and forgot to ask for a reward, as she had been accustomed to doing.

8

Typical Reactions to Specific Illnesses

So far as my own work was concerned, every child had to be dealt with as an individual, strictly on the basis of his own personal qualities and peculiarities. On the other hand, it would have been difficult not to take note of some typical behavioral reactions to specific forms of disease or specific modes of medical regime. The most striking among the latter were the differences between the orthopedic and the cardiac patients, in this instance in spite of the fact that the regimes were not dissimilar: as mentioned before, for both treatment started with immobilization which was gradually reduced as there was recovery of function.

ORTHOPEDIC PATIENTS

It was characteristic of the orthopedic patients that, with few exceptions, they accepted their confining and restricting treatments in a positive manner. They appeared content during immobilization, making a determined effort to bear their hardship and to improve their future physical condition. This attitude, which could be found even among the very young, was puzzling enough to arouse our curiosity and to make us search for explanations. There were several possible sources from which their surprising strength seemed to be derived.

First and foremost, the tangible and visible nature of the orthopedic devices seemed to be of help to them. There was no mystery anywhere, especially not in the information given. The various pieces of apparatus could be seen, examined, observed in action. So could the affliction itself, which was obvious in most instances. Treatment procedures could be discussed in definite and concrete terms, including the degree of improvement and the length of time needed for recovery; usually no sudden changes or relapses had to be feared in this respect. During their long-drawn-out convalescence, further knowledge about the mechanics of surgery, curiosity about X-rays, etc., provided a focus of interest for the older children. Somehow it seemed as if the stark and uncompromising reality of the situation, i.e., its very concreteness, served as reassurance and helped to keep fantasies and unrealistic anxieties in check.

Children in orthopedic treatment also derived strength from the group situation, i.e., from the realization that theirs was a common lot; that all of them had to submit to the same or similar restrictions; that most of them had for the time being lost the power of ambulation; that all of them were in the hospital to recover what they had lost.

Acceptance Based on Fantasy

On the other hand, unrealistic elements no less than the realistic ones seemed to play a role in the situation. What appeared as cheerful acquiescence on the surface often revealed itself on closer acquaintance with the child as the secret living out of masochistic or guilt-ridden attitudes. In connection with such tendencies children might experience the period of restrictive treatment as a time of suspense comparable to atonement, to be compared with the fairy tales where a happy ending is reached only after great hardship has been endured, such hardship not only being accepted but sought after and endowed with pleasurable anticipation.

DONNA[1] gave an example of this; she explained: "There are always three horrible tasks. One has first to find out what they are and then to fulfill them; only after one has suffered through it—only then can the prince or the princess return to his former shape." In her particular case, these tasks were represented by the two operations she had undergone and her wish for the magical third which would break the spell and restore her to health.

Other children, too, seemed to expect that miraculous things would happen if only they waited for them

[1] For further observations of this child, see Chapters 6 and 11.

patiently enough. They compared themselves with the gingerbread children in the fairy tale who also have to remain motionless—hopeful that the spell would soon be broken and allow them to leap into unrestricted freedom. Almost all of them, underneath, wished for magic which could result in an instantaneous and complete cure.

Breakdown of Acceptance

It was almost a relief for the observing adult that the children's strange contentment was not maintained under all circumstances. Above all it seemed to depend on everybody being treated alike and on everything happening according to plan; changes were not accepted easily.

Our children were known to react, for example, with severe temper tantrums and despair whenever any additional and unexpected measure had to be imposed on them, especially if this was not connected with their main affliction. Such situations caught them unprepared, off balance, and unwilling to cooperate.

Sixteen-year-old HENRY, for example, had experienced three major operations and, being a paraplegic, the treatment to improve his physical condition was extremely arduous. There was no comparison between these hardships and the little effort he would have to make to consent to having a broken tooth extracted. Yet, this he was unable to face and he insisted that he could not stand the thought of having one more injection. The latter was the door which opened up a flood of hitherto hidden feelings

REACTIONS TO SPECIFIC ILLNESSES 63

concerning his operations and the postoperative treatments. He himself could explain that under no circumstances would he enter any situation reminding him of these traumatic events and the accompanying fantasies. He knew quite well that sooner or later he would have to have this tooth removed since it was infected and very painful. However, at the moment he was neither willing nor able to accept any but his orthopedic physician's demands.

Another case was JOEL, who was five years old when he marched into our ward. He suffered from Legg-Perthes disease. He carried a bundle containing his favorite toys and belongings on his shoulder, acting like a soldier carrying his kit. He went around to greet all the children and then went quite happily to bed, where his legs were rested on a board raised at a considerable angle. He seemed happy, and not even during the first days of his stay did he mind the awkward position he was put in; he smiled and made friends with everyone. Every time his board was raised a bit higher, he proudly announced the fact and showed his extension weights the way he would have shown off a precious gift.

Yet this very child who was so proud of his extensions was terribly ashamed and unhappy when once he had to wear a bandage around his head because of an earache. He complained that with such a bandage he could do nothing. He covered his head with the sheet and lay in bed motionless. It was not pain which disturbed his play or work; he explicitly emphasized that the bandage around his head hampered him. What he did was to shift the blame for his handicap from the actual but accepted orthopedic device onto the bandage, which he experienced as disgraceful, extraordinary, and not belonging to the situation.[2]

Revolt during Recovery

Whereas during the immobilization period most children were overly patient and broke down only when additional discomfort was inflicted, they behaved quite differently when ambulation was begun. At this particular period of recovery, the behavior of the patients was for the most part characterized by general impatience and extreme sensitivity toward the slightest further restriction. Any treatment at this point was experienced as an insurmountable task and the seeming contentment, courage, and poise disappeared altogether. At times it was strange to see our formerly submissive and cooperative children changed into difficult patients, full of complaints and self-pity whenever a blood sample had to be taken or a splint applied. Evidently, after all the hardship they had undergone, they felt entitled to enjoy freedom to the full and were unwilling to be further imposed upon. Moreover, the magical expectations of quite a few children suffered severe relapses at the hand of reality at this time, owing to the unexpectedly slow progress in ambulation and the many remaining defects. Children who, at the time of approaching recovery, had joyfully anticipated "breaking the cast into smithereens" found

[2] This child was observed in England and described in greater detail by T. Bergmann: Observation of Children's Reactions to Motor Restraint. *Nerv. Child*, 4:318-328, 1945.

themselves still having to depend on braces, crutches, and so forth.

Reactions to Removal of Cast

It was also at this particular period of recovery that tension and anxiety broke through and found their outlet in aggression. With most of the active modes of discharge still blocked, rage usually revealed itself in temper tantrums and abusive language, both of unusual proportions, threatening to parents and not easy to deal with for the hospital staff. Luckily, such reactions were short lived and vanished again once a higher degree of motor function was restored.

It was instructive to experience that there were also children who reacted negatively to the shedding of casts and the recovery of freedom. In some instances the cast itself acted as a protective measure.

This happened with two adolescent girls, SYLVIA and LILY, who had developed a very close and intimate friendship which was primarily based on their similar situation: they felt that their casts in which they convalesced after spinal fusion were their "little houses," in which they lived as friendly neighbors—borrowing and sharing experiences, fantasies, and also doubts. "It's nice—you are snug in there, nobody can push you around," they commented. In the "snug little houses" they became almost defiant and they planned to stay this way.

Moreover, while in the cast, Sylvia had been prevented from giving in to masturbation, which she feared as "undesirable and not nice." The snug little house had protected her from conflicts which she formerly had had to face and which she dreaded in the future.

Another adolescent, GENE, became extremely upset when the time approached for his cast to be removed. He was a difficult postpolio patient, belligerent and moody. In his case, the cast did not prevent sexual excitement, but, on the contrary, made him "mad" when he had erections. He would then break out into abusive language, which the staff found hard to endure. Although he explained how glad he was "to get rid of the cast at long last," his attitude did not match such happy anticipation. On the contrary, his anxieties rose to a pitch and fastened on to the very procedure of cast removal, which he dreaded almost as if it were another operation. The fear of having his sexual manipulations discovered obviously was transformed into fear of "being cut by accident" by the blunt wheel used on the plaster of Paris.

The difficulty of abandoning immobilization as a passive, regressive situation was especially marked in the case of KEITH, a boy of five, with spina bifida, who had spent almost all his life in hospitals, and was in traction when I first met him. Ambulation was tried, and he was taught to walk with the help of two canes. However, most of the time he clung to a chair or table, not using his legs but dragging them along, making practically no progress. Because of this unsuccessful attempt to ambulate him, it was decided to put him back in traction. It was thought that he would be extremely unhappy and disappointed to be once again restricted. However, he did not seem to mind; rather, he was relieved by the renewed immobilization and settled contentedly in his bed.

Reactions to Specific Illnesses

Evidently, when trying to walk, Keith had realized that now he belonged nowhere, neither to the sheltered group of sick children nor to those who were successful in establishing free motion. Since the steps to secure independence seemed too arduous for him, he resigned himself to remaining with the sheltered group. He compensated for his failure in ambulating by developing extraordinary skills with his hands. He was successful in discovering new ways to use old toys, was very much admired by the other immobilized children because of this ingenuity, and was happy about his popularity with them—a situation which he preferred to other forms of activity.

Other Effects of Motor Restraint

It was also interesting to realize that, in many cases, a distinct inhibition of verbal expression went parallel with immobilization, as if the restraint enforced on children's limbs spread further and affected more highly differentiated motor functions. While young children often regressed in verbalization or, when just having learned to speak, lost the achievement altogether, older children occasionally became quite taciturn. Again, such losses were merely transitory. With the cast or other restrictive measures removed, verbalization reinstated itself.

This was the case with KATIE, four years old, who was in a plaster cast because of clubfeet. During the period of immobilization it was noticed that although she was very intelligent and used educational toys very well, she would only point to the ones she wished to have but would not ask for them. Her vocabulary became extremely limited and consisted of only a few words such as "mommy," "dadda," "doggie," and "by-by." Coinciding with the removal of the cast she suddenly reverted to her former self—speaking adequately in short sentences.

That removal of the cast and recovery of motor function can result in developmental spurts was shown also by the case of CRAIG, a six-year-old boy, who was considered to be mentally retarded. I met him after he had spent a year on a Bradford frame and was gradually returning to ambulation. At that time he was prone to temper tantrums, tore his bed linen, pajamas and clothes, and behaved in babyish ways. For weeks he kept walking with no other interest apparent. But once ambulation was established satisfactorily, to everybody's surprise he settled down in school, worked at his age level, and gave no further evidance of mental backwardness.

CARDIAC PATIENTS

Taking into account the fact that orthopedic patients are often "healthy" apart from their disabilities while cardiac patients are "ill" in the true sense of the word, and leaving aside individual similarities and differences, it is still worthy of note that none of the typical reactions observed in children under orthopedic treatment were present in the children with heart disease, who, in contrast, appeared depressed, discouraged, and in many instances outright hypochondriacal.

In the initial stage immediately after admission to the hospital, we experienced it as hardship that there was very little comforting information which we could give these patients, since the prognosis usually was less certain, the rate of progress less predictable, and the relapses frequent. The absence of formidable apparatus, instead of being reassuring, instead left the child in emptiness, with no outward trappings to which fears could be attached and nothing but a mysterious, internal ailment, difficult to verify. It was not easy to explain heart action, especially to the younger children, and the very vagueness of this concept usually aroused more fears and fantasies than it allayed. Their best clues for measuring the intensity of illness usually were, apart from the heartbeat, the successive alterations in therapy and medication, which all the children watched keenly.

Contrary to our experiences with orthopedic patients, we felt that the cardiac children profited little or not at all from the group situation. They observed and competed with each other, but in an unhealthy and unhelpful manner, using other children's state not as encouragement but as an illustration and demonstration of their own plight. If another child improved, they questioned enviously why this was not happening to them. If relapses occurred on the ward, they expected the same fate. Altogether, the presence and close proximity of other children with the same illness were instrumental only in raising their alarm.

In the absence of other tangible outside indications of their illness, our patients became overinvolved with their heartbeat, which they checked avidly. They became deeply concerned whether it was too loud, too fast, or irregular, and they identified any changes as signs of danger. To bring the heartbeat under control, and keep it in order, became their major concern.

An example of such concentration on the heartbeat was seen in ten-year-old LEAH, one of our chronic cases. She had displaced her preoccupation from the heart itself to a symbol representing it, i.e., a small alarm clock, which became her most prized possession and which she dutifully wound every evening to awaken the whole ward at 6 A.M. —much to the chagrin of the other girls. When she had to leave Rainbow for a few days to go to Babies' and Children's Hospital for catherization of the heart under sedation, she took the clock to our office for safekeeping. On her first morning away, before the operation, she phoned the nurse, to make sure that the clock had been wound. According to her fantasy, it was essential that the clock should continue to tick while she herself would be sedated and unable to attend to her own heartbeat.

Although not actually knowledgeable about the action of the heart itself, many of our children had come into contact with the fact of heart diseases before and knew of the possibly ominous consequences. They had seen an immediate relative, a friend of the family, or another child die from the same illness, had experienced loss, and—instead of looking forward hopefully—merely denied the same possible outcome in their own case.

On the whole, most of our cardiac children were compliant, sad patients, who did not exhibit their discomforts but insisted, on the contrary, that everything was fine with them. If not handled very carefully, their tendency was to withdraw from emotional contacts and to turn their interests inward, with body and heartbeat assuming the place which normally in a child's life is held by the important people in the outside world.

9

Some Reactions to Other Afflictions

In spite of frequent visiting by parents and Sunday picnics with siblings, the significant social group for our children was the ward which during their long hospitalization replaced their home and school community. On the wards there was intense participation in the experiences important to other patients; knowledge of and keen interest in the others' afflictions and prognosis; acute observations in connection with improvements and recovery. In the comparative seclusion and inactivity of hospital life, the children interacted with each other and influenced each other to a degree not easily equaled in any other situation. Individual fears, hopes, and fantasies spread through the ward and were acted on even by children in whom they did not originate, a sharing of experience which was most intense, of course, where the affliction was the same.

It was inevitable, on the other hand, owing to hospital policy, that our children also met others whose illnesses were entirely new and strange to them and whose precarious state aroused further fears and fantasies with which we tried to deal.

THE IMPACT OF BLINDNESS

Few children have actually come in contact with a blind person, but for many blindness as a notion plays a part in their fantasy world as a symbol of severe body damage, i.e., castration. Nevertheless, there is a great difference between meeting in a classical saga the figure of the blind hero, punished by the gods, and actually living in the intimacy of the ward with a child who has lost his eyesight. Both occasions are frightening to the seeing child, but the latter acts as a greater shock, especially to children whose own bodily integrity is threatened by severe illness.

ROBERT, aged fourteen, was blind and deaf following an acute episode of sarcoidosis when he was admitted to our Boys' Ward for convalescence. Communication with him was restricted to writing on the palm of his hand. We prepared the boys simply by explaining to them that such unfortunate situations do exist, that there are people far more handicapped than they were themselves, and that they were going to have such a child in their midst; that it was up to them to conquer their anxieties about it and to be helpful to the newcomer.

Actually, we never knew whether our children coped so satisfactorily with the fears aroused in them, or whether it was simply Robert's disarmingly free and friendly disposition that bridged the abyss between him and the other children. Robert would openly say, "I cannot do that because I cannot see," or "This will take time for me to do because I am blind." The children adopted, quite ingeniously, some kinds of signs to communicate and then we heard Robert say, "Do not lead me—I have to find my way myself, but if you have time, will you walk with me?" They were very helpful to one another. Robert made many presents—these were beautiful lamps which he wired carefully and demonstrated proudly, enjoying the admiration of children and adults alike. It is interesting that Robert came to learn to build lamps to such perfection and that it was so important for him to provide light for his friends and to present them with something that he himself was denied.

But, in any case, the experiment worked and Robert became an accepted member of the group in spite of his deviant affliction.

THE IMPACT OF AMPUTATION

Since we found that the boys had been helped in coping with the situation by merely having their thoughts clarified and by having their questions answered openly and realistically, the same method was decided on when Connie's admission to Rainbow was discussed.

CONNIE had had one of her legs amputated as a small infant because of a tumor. When she was two and a half years old she was hospitalized at Rainbow to obtain a prosthesis and learn to walk.

We had to decide where to place her; while Connie, according to her age, belonged with the children on the Nursery Ward, we were reluctant to expose such young children to a one-legged newcomer. At this time of life castration fears are uppermost in all children and we did not think that our small patients, disturbed by their own shortcomings as they were, were in any way equipped to deal with the additional experience. Therefore, we opted for the Girls' Ward, with children from seven to twelve years, where the child's predicament could be discussed openly with the group, and separately with each child.

After JOYCE (Chapter 13) had been informed about Connie's condition, she called softly to me, "Come here— you mean they cut it off—just like that? [She made the gesture with her hand.] You mean they knew the leg was no good—huh? And there is no other growing? How does the baby feel about it? I sure would not want that to happen to me. They do not cut a leg off because of arthritis, do they?" She received assurance, but she persisted, "They might, though; I could be in a car accident. Well, I won't."

DIANA, a twelve-year-old paraplegic, was most sympathetic. "Just think, a little child growing up with only one leg and never knowing how it is to have two!" Diana cared for this little girl as if she were a precious doll, one that by a miracle was going to walk with one leg. She watched the achievements of this little child with great enjoyment and still greater sympathy, as if Connie were a broken toy which never could be repaired properly.

Connie stayed only a short while at Rainbow and although she was treated by all the children like the lovable little child she was, one could almost hear a sigh of relief when she left.

For us it was instructive to observe and discuss the children's reactions and to measure the distance which they felt existed between the severe impairment of their bodies or even complete loss of function of limbs and the actual loss of a limb. We wondered whether Diana, for example, realized that she would never walk in spite of possessing her two legs, whereas the "little broken doll" would soon move about on her prosthesis.

It was also of interest to us that Robert's defects were easier for the other children to accept than Connie's. Even if Robert could not see and hear, he had eyes and ears, as they had legs and arms which they could not use. Above all, he *looked* like them, and the absence of visible outward difference made sympathetic identification with him more feasible. In Connie's case, identification with her affliction was out of the question and all that the girls could fall back on as helpful defenses were a motherly, protective attitude toward her and pride in her achievements.

THE IMPACT OF DEATH

In Rainbow, a convalescent hospital, the children were usually spared the experience of losing their friends through death. When severe relapses occurred, the patients were transferred to Babies' and Children's Hospital before the fatal outcome. Such transfers happened frequently, for a variety of reasons, and the children were not concerned about them. They knew that such patients either would return to Rainbow after an interval or might be discharged from Babies' and Children's Hospital directly to their homes. They were equally prepared therefore for seeing them or not seeing them again.

The death of SAMMY, aged eleven, was for these reasons an unusual occurrence. Sammy, who suffered from muscular dystrophy, had felt worse one day, and arrangements were made to transfer him to Babies' and Children's Hospital next morning. However, before his transfer could be arranged, he suddenly died.

As was customary when a patient was examined on the ward, the curtains around Sammy's bed were drawn. The nurse in charge told the children that the doctor wanted to have it quiet in the ward for Sammy's sake and she sent them off to me, to play. They left in a strange hurry, excited, noisy, and giggling. While they were with me, they played and acted in a mood of high elation as if they were attending a successful party—a state of mind not unusual for children under tragic circumstances of this kind. By the time they returned for lunch, Sammy had left the ward.

According to hospital routine, the nurses had done their best to protect their patients and to avoid arousing their anxieties. Nevertheless, they themselves felt upset about Sammy's death and the other children undoubtedly sensed their feelings. They began to collect money to send flowers to Sammy, although usually it would never have occurred to them to give a parting present to a patient about to be transferred elsewhere. This unusual reaction in itself was a sign that they had guessed the truth.

Personally, I felt very doubtful whether their intention would be carried out, and events proved me right; the forty-seven cents which they had collected disappeared mysteriously during the rest period and nobody seemed eager to try and find the money. Perhaps the children felt that they had paid their tribute and the intention in itself was sufficient to relieve anxiety.

If accused of not having been honest with the children on the occasion of Sammy's death, we would have had to plead guilty. Probably, if a child had asked outright, my answer would have been a truthful one, but nobody did ask the question and I felt reluctant to volunteer the information. Sammy, who had died of muscular dystrophy, was not the only patient with this affliction in the ward. There seemed no point in alerting his fellow patients to the possibility that the same fatal outcome might be in store for them.

Altogether, it is difficult to imagine any way in which one could prepare a child for death, either that of a fellow patient or his own. For the children themselves, death has little meaning apart from the idea of "being away," "gone." For the adults who have to watch it, the death of a young child remains an event against nature, an experience which many find almost beyond acceptance.

Whenever a child is destined to die on the ward, and especially when deterioration is slow and of long duration, the question arises for the adults how to act toward him, because neither honesty nor reassurance even remotely meets the situation. The only answer we could find was to help the child to live through all his ups and downs fully and in the ordinary way while life is there, i.e., to deal with every incidence of his illness, including deterioration, as a part of life which has to be met as such, not as a preparation for death. Probably, the only way in which the child spontaneously grasps the notion of death is—if not through the parents' upset—via the feeling of tiredness and the disinclination to make further efforts. All that is left for the adult to do then is to permit the child increasingly to give in to this negative desire.

10

Illness Misunderstood as Punishment

There is in many children's minds, a firmly fixed belief that illnesses are self-induced, the well-deserved punishment for all sorts of badness, disobedience, disregard of rules, neglect of prohibitions, bodily abuse. Parental warnings against foolhardiness and self-indulgence, cautionary tales, and religious teachings about sin and retribution, wherever they occur, give authoritative backing to these convictions, which are rooted in guilt about the common sexual-aggressive impulses of childhood and their discharge in masturbation. While such mistaken notions, even though upsetting, may remain of minor significance for the bodily healthy child, they become important to the severely ill, since they sap the child's strength to fight his disease by creating a false, masochistic, and morbidly accepting attitude toward suffering.

Illness as Punishment

In the hospital, we became familiar with this idea of "badness," which cropped up repeatedly and in a variety of ways.

ERNEST, an attractive eight-year-old boy, in the hospital after an attack of rheumatic fever with signs of chorea, regarded hospitalization and treatment as a result of having been "bad." Probably on the strength of this, he was quiet and obedient.

He confided to me how upset he was about two boys in the ward who exhibited sexual play. They were as bad, he stated, as the children on the street with whom he had played before his illness. He did not want to have anything more to do with them, because what they did "was bad and dangerous." After that the following conversation took place between us:

I asked, "What is bad and dangerous?"
Ernest: "To play with it."
"Why should it be dangerous?"
"Because it's dangerous to touch it, because you can get germs on it."
"Where do you get germs?"
"On my hands."
"Would they harm you on your hands?"
"No, but if I touch it with my hands the germs could get on it."
"Why should germs be more harmful on another part of the body than on hands?"
"I don't know, but one should not touch it because the germs can make you sick."
"All children touch it and do not get sick from it. If they get sick, it is not because of that—and you are not sick because you touched it. What is really the name of 'it'?"

"I don't know."
"What do the boys on the ward call it?"
"Wiener."
"Do you say Wiener too?"
"Yes."
"That is the name many little children use. Grownups call it "penis."
This frightened Ernest all the more and he said in bewilderment: "Penis? You said it was penis? But then one does get sick from touching it, because Gary touched it and he got sick, and they gave him *peni*cillin."

Ernest's preoccupation with the similarity between the words "penis" and "penicillin," which to the adult sounds almost like a pun, is in fact a serious matter for this child. Children with rheumatic fever live under the constant threat of infection and much of their treatment is centered around the effort to avoid infection. Even the pulling of a tooth requires the precaution of a penicillin injection, since any infection may cause a severe relapse. While, on the one hand, such children acquire ample realistic knowledge about such medical precautions, on the other hand, their fantasies and masturbation guilt run riot concerning the same subjects.

RUTH, aged nine, came to Rainbow with rheumatic heart disease for which she had to observe complete bed rest. She was entirely uncomplaining. She told us that she had always tried to be the "goodest" of the four children in her family because "Mother and the Lord are always aware of children's sins." Sometimes she had been bad too, but not like the boys, and yet it was she who had become sick, a

ILLNESS AS PUNISHMENT

fact which she considered as unfair. She was worried by the memory that she had masturbated and that then her heart had begun "pounding," and she thought this the reason that she had a bad heart. Talking about it to me seemed to relieve her conscience temporarily and to calm her.

Our conversations were taken up again when I had to prepare her for tonsillectomy which she faced composedly except for the fear of "talking while asleep" and "giving away" whatever she thought. She was reassured again that masturbation had not made her ill and that she probably would not talk under the anesthetic, especially if she ceased worrying. However, instead of allaying her fears, my reassurances were taken as seduction to badness and treated as such. She returned to Rainbow in a hostile mood, telling me that her father had been with her before surgery and had taught her not to be afraid, that the Lord would be with her and protect her if she had no sins. Accordingly, she had decided never to sin again and, protected by the Lord, she would never be ill again.

"Badness" also played a major part in the case of CINDY, aged four and a half, hospitalized because of Guillain-Barré syndrome. She was a difficult patient, probably owing to a traumatic syringing of her ears at three, in connection with which she had suffered severe pain and a swollen face. Since then she had had an intense fear of doctors and, according to her parents' report, became panicky at every medical visit or injection, so that "they could hardly hold her down because she fought like mad and screamed that she always would be good if only nothing was done to her."

Cindy was a clever and beautiful little girl, born to her

parents after sixteen years of marriage. Although delighted with her initially, they had become worried about and discouraged by her aggressive behavior and punished her severely, which did not help matters. The father said repeatedly: "She is bad, she is really bad." Cindy herself repeated, often and quite freely, that she was sick and had to stay in the hospital because she was "a bad girl."

Actually, in the hospital Cindy's behavior varied, and she displayed both positive and negative attitudes. After a session with me, when I presented her with some game or handiwork to finish on the ward, she would say gratefully: "Thank you, thank you, thank you very much, this will keep me busy and out of mischief." At other times she would act out her hostility against her mother in play, stuffing a mother doll forcibly into a little buggy and saying: "Mothers can be sick. She can sit in the buggy. She can be in the hospital." She also explained that "always, always" she had to fight—her boy friend because he teased her, ghosts "because they are after you when you are bad." Once, after she had pushed her bed near a very sick, helpless baby and thrown a pillow over his face, she explained that she could not stand his crying. She had to fight the children on the ward, she said, because they frightened her. "They scare me. They are very sick and I will get more sick from them. . . . I got sick from another bad child because *I* am bad. The baby is very sick and he is very bad, he cries all the time." Cindy had learned about contagion at a time when she had to be isolated for infection. But in her mind illness and "badness" had become hopelessly confused, so that children who were sicker than she was had to be fought off as bad, "contagious" influences.

Another instance of the same confusion was presented by ELIZABETH, ten and a half years old. Suffering from acute rheumatic fever, she was tall, somewhat obese, quiet and bashful, soft-spoken, well behaved, and uncomplaining. Her mother, widowed since the death of her alcoholic husband, had had to place the four children in foster homes. Elizabeth herself had been fostered by a devoted elderly Italian couple for some years and professed to resemble her foster mother, which in fact she did. Nevertheless she was in a conflict of loyalty to her real mother and her foster mother, had unrealistic expectations of being taken "home" by her real mother, and claimed that she would never have fallen ill under her own mother's care, etc.

After some time on the ward it was reported that Elizabeth had become increasingly restless and unhappy. This was attributed to the lack of improvement in her condition. In actuality, however, it turned out that her complaints were directed against another girl on the ward of whom she had initially been fond. This girl, helpless herself, demanded assistance, to which Elizabeth reacted excitedly: "I cannot. I am not supposed to and it harms me." Or, when her friend wanted to talk in the evening: "I cannot. I am not supposed to, and she gets mad at me if I try to go to sleep. If I talk, I cannot rest, and I will not get better."

After consulting with both girls, their beds were separated; thereupon it proved to be impossible to find the right place to suit Elizabeth. She was afraid to see a window at night; she was afraid to hear the rain; she could not bear to see the lightning if there was a storm; the shadows of the branches frightened her when they moved, etc.

Next, she confided to me that she was always afraid the shadow might be that of a man. She never went out alone any more in the dark, she said, since she had been followed by a man who exhibited in front of her. "If I look out of a window and I see a shadow, I *have* to keep looking at it and it reminds me of it and I get so upset and then my heart beats fast. That's why I am not getting better." Similarly, she described her excitement when listening to mysteries over the radio. "I hate it, but then I *have* to listen all the time. I have to think of that man, and I get more and more excited and my heart beats faster and faster. I know I should not listen to it because of my heart, but then I can't give it up."

It was known on the ward that Elizabeth's friend masturbated excessively and she herself admitted that she too "a long time ago" had done the same. "Does one get a weak heart if one makes it beat so fast? The trouble is that I do not take it easy, because I can't give up the radio because I like it so much. And when I listen, I get upset and afraid of it."

In the meantime Elizabeth became able to go to school, but she was not yet allowed uptime because of her high sedimentation rate. In her talks with me she next expressed her concern about menstruation, i.e., the notion of "bad blood" which had to be lost in menstruation. Would she be able ever to lose bad blood? She was afraid of having a blood sample taken, but not of the pain involved. "No," she said, "that's not it. I hate it because I do not know what they want to find out about my blood. Can they find out whether blood is bad?"

I reminded her that I had told her before that there is no such thing as "bad blood." We also discussed again the procedure of taking a sample of blood in order to determine the sedimentation rate.

Elizabeth insisted that people could find out other things than the sedimentation rate and that worried her. She told about a newspaper article of which she had heard, which had stated that one could find out by looking at blood samples whether a person is the father of a baby. She asked, "Is it true that one could find that the father had the same blood as the baby?"

I explained that this was correct—that certain blood consistencies could prove that.

Elizabeth asked, "If the father had bad blood, would the child have it too?"

Finally, her underlying worry emerged. She had learned in school that Indians were bad, having killed white people. "They have red skin and that comes from their blood which is different from that of white people. My father was Indian—but I do not want anybody to know that I had a bad father. Could they find out from my blood?" Obviously, she had often heard her father being called "bad" because of his drunkenness.

With this revelation of her "guilty secret" and my reassurances (that Indians are no worse than the whites, that killing happened whenever there was fighting, that no one could find out her Indian parentage, but that it would not matter if they did, etc.) Elizabeth began to settle down. She stressed again her looking like an Italian girl, i.e., a "good" person, wanting to be "good" herself on all accounts. But she also became more relaxed and outgoing—and, interesting enough, her sedimentation rate came down rapidly for the first time. Even before it was at the normal level, she was considered well enough to be discharged.

I heard later that she became quite confident and mature in her behavior and that her foster parents took great pride and pleasure in her.

11

Denials, Regressions, Other Defensive Devices, and Constructive Resources

While all children during their personality development are confronted by external and internal dangers and learn to cope with them by means of their defenses, our young patients were challenged in addition by chronic illness, the implied threats to health and life, as well as by pain, frustration, deprivation. No wonder that their resources were taxed to the utmost and not always equal to the task. When coming to their help, on the other hand, their own methods and devices had to be respected. While a physically healthy child in psychotherapy can be deprived of primitive denial, withstand anxiety, and be expected to resort to more mature defenses subsequently, the balance which the chronically ill have created for themselves is extremely subtle and precarious. If forced to meet excessive anxiety undefended, the child may be thrown merely into stark despair and hopelessness. For this reason the approach used was to follow the child on the path he had adopted for himself, to adapt to his adjustments, to help him to overcome obstacles and elucidate anxieties in his own way, and to allow a new and less distorted view of the situation to emerge very slowly, with as little disturbance as possible.

DENIAL AND NIGHTMARES

BETTY, a ten-year-old girl, contracted bulbar polio while on vacation and became desperately ill; for most of the first year after the onset of her illness she was completely paralyzed, lived in a respirator, and for a long time remained on the danger list. Because transportation to a hospital closer to her home was impossible, the mother decided to work as a hospital aide to be near the child. She stated that Betty had been the most favored patient during her long acute phase because her cheerfulness and determination to get well were an inspiration to everyone. She was most helpful with other children and often successful in achieving their cooperation where others failed.

When Betty came to Rainbow, the characterization given by the mother was fully confirmed. She was a charming child, made friends easily, and nothing seemed to worry her. Instead she said: "Isn't it a miracle how well I am?" By this time she had almost completely recovered her muscle power and moved around gracefully. Only one handicap remained: she could not use the muscles of her eyes and therefore had to move her head in a peculiar

Defenses and Constructive Resources 91

way. Her own ego strength very likely was the reason for "the miracle to be so well."

Although Betty did extremely well during the day, she began to suffer from nightmares during which she screamed. The fears which she had so successfully denied when they were real and at their height in the acute stage of her illness she relived now in her dreams. She was very apologetic about the "noise" she made and feared that the girls would like her less because she was disturbing them with her "silly screaming."

I explained to her that she might be able to stop the screaming if she could recall her dreams and find out what really worried her. However, for quite a while she insisted that she had no dreams, that nothing worried her, and that she felt well. After some time, though, she came to report with a shy little laugh that she had screamed again and this time she remembered her dream. However, she could not believe that a dream as silly as that could make her scream. She said:

> I was in the bathtub. I wanted to get out, but could not. I called my mommy. She did not come. I screamed and screamed. That is all.
>
> Why should I be afraid of a bathtub? When I was in the hospital I never was so afraid. I wasn't as afraid as I was in the bathtub. I knew what was going on in the hospital. I helped everybody. I helped all the children. I helped Ruth. She would only eat for me. When you come out of the respirator you think you have to die, you can stay out only for one minute. You cannot breathe. You get used to it. I am so well because my doctor knew and let me out only for one minute until

I got used to it. I helped Ruth. She did not know
—she was only four.

Here her voice became louder and louder, and finally, almost screaming, she told how little Ruth was taken out of the respirator one night and she knew that Ruth could not live that long out of it and she knew therefore that her little friend had died. Everybody tried to tell her that this was not so, but finally, probably screaming, as she had done at night, she said, "Nobody can fool me. I know she was dead and I can't understand why it is that I am alive." She added that she would become a children's doctor or a nurse when she grew up, because she knew what it was like to be afraid, to fear dying, not to be able to "do anything for yourself."

This was probably the first time that Betty had permitted herself to cry desperately about the loss of her little friend and also allowed herself to face her very own anxiety, namely, the fact that she had been in the same danger. Betty did not suffer from any further nightmares for the remaining time she spent at Rainbow. But interestingly, she did not like it at Rainbow any more and, while quite satisfied and happy only a short time before, she now began to find fault, became critical, and created difficulties between staff and parents. Disagreeable as it was for the personnel to handle these upsets, for Betty herself it was an important step to uncover some of the anxieties she had been unable to recognize before. The repression of her emotions and denial of her anxiety had made it possible for her to become the perfect patient and to settle down so well in the hospital. Now that the defenses of repression and denial had been rendered ineffective, she also became aware of her dislike of being hospitalized and her dissatisfaction with the shortcomings of hospital life.

DENIAL BY FANTASY

SOPHIA, a very pretty thirteen-year-old Negro girl, had been in a body cast for almost six months following a spinal fusion, when she drew a picture portraying herself as a beautiful blonde dancer. Although the fantasy could not have been further removed from the truth, still it helped her to accept the frustrating reality of her situation.

WITHDRAWAL AND REVERSAL

DONNA,[1] aged ten, afflicted with tuberculosis of the spine, experienced many traumatic procedures during her long hospitalization. Gradually, she changed from a lively, outgoing child who had been the leader on her ward, to a quiet, withdrawn, submissive patient who lost all interest in anything except her illness. As her condition became worse, it became necessary to isolate her. She probably sensed the sympathy and concern that she awakened, and then she reversed the role of concern and was most solicitous in advising others to take good care of themselves by following the rules of isolation. "You have to wear a gown, you have to wash your hands," she would advise her visitors. In this way she succeeded in turning away from her concern about herself and from the anxieties engendered by her condition. She emphasized that she was happy—she preferred to be alone and apart from all that previously had been important to her. She was determined to become a nun and she explained, "It is better to live the

---

[1] For further material on Donna, see Chapters 6 and 8.

hard way. A nun cannot go out, she has to sleep on a hard bed, and she has to work hard. She has to live without father and mother. When you live the hard way, then the Lord will be with you."

No purpose would have been served by disturbing the child in her primitive reversal of affect. By demonstrating "This is what I want, this is what I myself chose," she could feel that she was mastering her own fate and gather the strength to bear the hardship which was imposed on her.

ADAPTATION BY REGRESSION

There are other forms of adaptation to illness which are too damaging to the child's progress to be left uninterfered with. Foremost among these are the regressive moves made by ill children.

When HARRIET,[2] aged ten, was afflicted with extremely severe polio, she was able to enjoy care for the first time in her life. Neglected by her own mother, she had been placed in a foster home at the age of five months and since then had made the rounds of many homes, unable to settle down anywhere. While severely sick and handicapped she slipped back into the passive helplessness of an infant; as such she was easy to nurse and in good contact with the staff. During her convalescence in Rainbow, where more activity and independence were expected from her, she felt lost and forlorn again, and returned to the sullen unhappiness of earlier times.

In her case, there were many indications that she was ready to sacrifice physical improvement for the sake of

[2] See also Chapter 7.

enjoyable dependence; therefore, with her, the task was to coax her gradually to renounce this incapacitating regression.

AN EXAMPLE OF MASTERY

DAVE, aged nine, gave an excellent example of constructive reversal of affect, resignation, insight, and mastery by means of wit and humor. When he began his convalescence from poliomyelitis at Rainbow, there was still extensive involvement of his whole body and he was quite frail. He was fully aware of the danger he was in and able to meet his feelings even though he belittled them. His story is given best in his own words in the form of an autobiographical sketch written at age eleven, i.e., two years after the onset of illness:

LOG OF MY LIFE

I was born in New Orleans, Louisiana, on September 15, 1943. Dad had just been discharged from the Air Corps and he went to Berkeley, California, to teach in the medical school there. Mother and I stayed in Louisiana until he found a place for us to live. There was a bayou in back of our house. Mom and I used to go down there to gather pecans; we didn't know until later that there were coral snakes back there.

When I was three, we moved to Medina, Ohio. We lived in town until I had finished the first grade; then we moved to the house where we are still living. There is a big pine in back of our house that I used to love to climb, especially on windy days. Tony [a friend] and I used to wrestle, and he could always get me with a "Boston Crab." One day when he had it "on" me, I kicked out and sent his 175 pounds rocketing into a rose bed. One night Tony and I camped out; he had to go to a Boy Scout meeting and I kept the fire going for four hours. It was fun being alone with no company except for an occasional airplane.

On May 12, 1951, we adopted a six-month-old baby girl who was to become known to the world as Deborah. About a month later we adopted a three-month-old Dachshund who was to become known to the world as Duchess von Vickie.

On Wednesday, July 13, 1952, I got polio. I had had a pain in my back ever since Monday. That day I was out rowing with Tony and I had to vomit. I asked him to put me on shore, and when he did I ran up to the house. I think that is probably the last time I ever ran. Within an hour I was "booked" in the Medina Hospital. I was charged with having polio. I had to plead guilty, and my sentence was life imprisonment in a wheel chair. When I was in the respirator, in a coma, the only thing I remember is getting plasma through a little hole in the top of the respirator. During those days in the respirator the only recreation was trying to blow at a balloon that my folks had brought me that was fixed over my head. One of the worst things that I remember is that when I couldn't talk for a while, and because I couldn't call for water, I got thirstier than I ever have been. I was in the respirator for about six weeks. At the end of that time I got out into a bed in a semiprivate room. I remember that I thought my roommate was a sissy because he wore pink glasses.

I had a week end at home when I left the Medina Hospital. We had gotten a TV set while I was in the hospital and I watched everything on it. When the allotted week end was up, I went to Rainbow Hospital. I celebrated my birthday by getting up for the first time since I'd been sick. I got a bad cold and was sent to Babies' and Children's Hospital (commonly referred to as B. & C.). I spent Christmas there. They allowed Debbie to come up to see me for that one day. I went back to Rainbow and stayed there until I went to another convalescent hospital, which was closer to home, early in April.

It would take a book to tell everything that happened to me there. The most exciting thing that happened while I was there was the "WAR" and its aftermath. One night one of the night watchmen saw a light burning in one of the young Negro orderly's rooms. He walked in and found one of the more studious Negroes studying late. He did not like this and he beat the Negro. He was allowed to go free because he was white and his victim was black. That's very fine justice, isn't it?

One Negro, Mr. M., who gave us our baths, was enraged about it. He said that he was going to catch the night watchman and beat him up. He ambushed him one night and everybody was surprised because Mr. M. was the most peaceful fellow that you could hope to meet. I don't know what happened to him.

I stayed at this convalescent hospital for about six months. At the end of this time I went home. I had my fifth-grade work over a telephone intercommunication system connected with Kingston School. I went back to Dr. H., an orthopedic surgeon at the hospital in Cleveland. He had taken care of me before when I was in Cleveland. He said that my feet should be operated on and also my hands. So I went to B. & C. and Dr. H. operated on my feet (which turned out all right). Another doctor "did" my hand (which wasn't successful). I went home for a while until it was time for my casts to come off. After they were taken off at B. & C., I went to Rainbow again.

Rainbow had the best food of any hospital I've ever been in. My physical therapist was Mrs. K. She was one of the best in the business. The nurse in the daytime was Miss T. She was a corker. She was a perfect example of a nurse. She wouldn't pay attention to what you had to say—she just went right ahead and did what she pleased while you yelled bloody murder. They had a grand library there. It must have had two or three thousand books in it. They had regular classes at Rainbow. All the pupils in the sixth grade were boys at this time!

I finally came home where I have been for about a year. The main thing that I remember was our vacation last summer in New York. My aunt teaches in a college and we went to visit her. We took trips all over New York, Vermont, and New Hampshire. I organized the R.E.C. [Recreation-Exploration Club], which is probably the only official one of its kind in the country. We came back after a month and in September I started going to school for half a day. I am in the seventh grade. A certain Mr. N. became our teacher. He's the one who gave me this darned autobiography to write, and now it's finished.

Although most feelings, especially sadness, were kept fully in check in Dave's autobiography, significantly enough, one affect broke through and was expressed fully: his resentment of injustice. Discriminated against like the young Negro, he was "sentenced to life imprisonment in a wheel chair," a procedure regarded by him as "fine justice."

All that Dave had after rehabilitation were the use of the right arm and hand—and these were weakened —a good mind, a lively sense of humor, great pleasure in reading, and enjoyment of life as far as possible under these circumstances. He died, aged fifteen, following the second of two operations planned to correct curvature of the spine due to polio.

12

Illness and Personality Development

There is, perhaps, no place where the interaction between body and mind can be studied more advantageously than in a hospital for chronically ill children. What we saw demonstrated to the full was how in some instances personality development can be distorted and devastated by the affliction of the body; how in others a strong ego may triumph over the body, influence progress and recuperation, and mold the final outcome; and, finally, how helplessly exposed to their illnesses were those children whose earlier circumstances of life had deprived them of the chance of building up healthy and effective personalities. In what follows I chose three specific cases as particularly impressive illustrations: Stephen for succumbing to his illness, Carl for dominating it, and Larry as a child who had to be helped in the hospital to develop controls and defenses which more fortunate children acquire in the intimacy of the family situation.

PHYSICAL ILLNESS AS A DESTRUCTIVE FORCE

STEPHEN, aged six, had entered the hospital after an upsetting incident during rough play when he kicked a mentally deficient boy (also called Stephen) who promptly had convulsions. As punishment he was confined to the house for the following week, during which he himself developed polio. How far anxiety, guilt, distress due to the coincidence of the two events heightened his fears and made him regard his illness as punishment remained unknown to us.

In any case, Stephen was a very submissive and good patient in the acute phase, but while convalescing at Rainbow he acted strangely, was considered immature and withdrawn, and did not enjoy the company of others. He did not seem to understand what was said, or forgot it on the spot, spilled his drinks and his urinal, kicked and struck the adults who handled him. "Then I get madder and madder and madder," as he explained himself. At nighttime he did not use a soft toy to help him go to sleep but had to have a cowboy hat instead. In anxiety he clutched his penis. Once, after an aggressive outbreak against another child, when I explained to him that I thought it unfair of him to hit Mark, who was three years younger and could not defend himself against a bigger, stronger boy, he said: "You say I am strong? They always say I have to lie down because I am weak. Mark is sick like I am and he can walk."

Stephen's polio was less extensive than others' and

medically the outlook for his recovery was good. Nevertheless, unlike others, he was concerned with the thought of death. "Could a car fall off a jack? Would people die in it? Could a little doll 'slip' and die in the bathtub? Can one have measles twice? Can one die because of measles? Can one have polio twice?"—and finally, "Can one die of polio?" When told by his parents about President Roosevelt's achievements in spite of polio, he asked whether Roosevelt was still president; when told he was dead, came the question: "Did he die of polio?"

At the parents' request I kept in touch with Stephen after his discharge because of the numerous difficulties that they were unable to deal with. I tried to help the child while urging the parents to seek analytic treatment for him.

First, wearing braces and limping only slightly, Stephen attended a school for crippled children, but he was so badly frightened by the severe handicaps of the others that he had temper tantrums of the worst sort.

In public school, which he attended next, he was a failure in spite of a recorded I.Q. of 175 (!). His work was extremely untidy and to prevent his parents from seeing it, he "lost" his books on the way home. Actually, he admitted to me that he threw the books into the bushes so that he could run faster. I reminded him that nobody could run very fast while wearing braces and for a time he would have to let the others win in this respect; however, we knew he could run much faster than anyone else in his class as far as work, especially reading, was concerned. "Yeah," he said, "there you have something, but I have to run fast, I have to run like the others, I have to run *faster*."

At the same time it became almost an obsession with

him to draw and study electrical appliances—to study what makes things "go" and "run." When I pointed out to him that all the wires in his excellent sketches looked like muscles which also make things run and go, he answered, "Yeah, that's why it's so interesting."

When he wrote about electricity, I offered to spell this difficult word for him, but he explained: "Everybody knows 'elect' like elect a president, everybody knows how to spell 'city,' all you have to do is put 'ri' in between.

"Electricity was known 2,000 years ago. The Greek people found a stone which they called an electron. When they rubbed it they felt something like a current. That's why it is called electricity. It was very weak. Now electricity is very powerful. *It can kill people.*"

Once when Stephen was punished in school and had to remain behind in order to finish his schoolwork, he wrote the following essay:

ENGINES

There are several types of engines. I am going to discuss gas, diesel, and steam engines. Gas engines have four steps. They are: (1) intake, (2) compression, (3) power, and (4) exhaust. A gas engine consists of a cylinder, a piston, a crank, a crankshaft.

Intake—a gas and air mixture is drawn into the cylinder.

Compression—piston compresses the gas.

Power—the spark plug explodes the gas, producing power.

Exhaust—burned gas is exhausted from the cylinder. The exhaust gases are CO, a very poisonous gas. If an automobile was running in a closed garage with a man in the garage, *the man would be dead.*

Stephen then went on to discuss steam, diesel, and atomic engines in the same manner. At the age of ten he became equally absorbed in the notion of atomic power —the complete destruction of everything. His knowledge, then, was comparable to that of a college student, and it became impossible for me to follow his drawings, which, incidentally, were found to be accurate by others. His father, himself an electrical engineer, blamed himself for having set the child off on this path but admitted that the boy's unusual proficiency fascinated him.

As he previously had had to run like others, and had to run faster, he now had to *know*—"But I have to *know more.*" It seemed that he was driven to know all or even "more" about this particular subject because he desired so vehemently to be protected against atomic power—protected against his own destructive forces. Yet, by using his outstanding intelligence, he actually never appeared conflicted, and he was unable to accept guidance—the more so because this particular and strange ability earned him a great deal of satisfying admiration.

In spite of his brilliance, he performed poorly in school and only made passing grades if given the utmost consideration. His relationships to teacher and children, particularly his abusive speech and disturbed manners, even led to his temporary expulsion from school, which was a great shock to him and resulted in a very brief improvement upon his return.

My interviews with the parents were rewarding in so far as they accepted some explanations of Stephen's conflicts, became less harsh and punishing in their attitude and more protective and tactful in handling the school situation. Still, Stephen remained a lonely child, dominated by anxieties which he denied, outstandingly brilliant, without friends, and sharing few interests with his two younger brothers. Although he learned to some extent to cope with his aggression, especially at home, his problems in school remained frequent and his performance was poor.

There were two subsequent corrective operations during which he behaved, according to the nurse's report, like "a real little gentleman"—probably because he was paralyzed by fear.

At the age of twelve he met with a fatal accident. He had left the basement in disorder and as punishment was sent down to clean up. Two hours later he was found, strangled, with an electric cord around his neck. Whether this was accidental or a deliberate suicidal attempt remained unsolved. In any case, his fantasy that "electricity is powerful, it can kill people" had found its realization in fact.

It would be erroneous, of course, to contend that Stephen's conflicts, his difficult character structure, and other abnormalities had been *created* by his chronic illness. The same clashes between a highly organized ego on the one hand and the sexual-aggressive impulses on the other hand occur in many children, physically ill or healthy. Furthermore, the fears of retribution and the anxiety attacks, the inhibitions in school performance and adaptation, the defensive use of his outstanding brilliance in selected areas, the turning of aggression against the self—all these are well known to every student of childhood neuroses, and are commonly overcome by the child, either with or without therapeutic help. What created the difference in Stephen's case and rendered him unable either to cope on his own or to accept help was a specific aspect of the matter. With the physically healthy child, the fears of castration, death, and annihilation are products of his fantasy, recognized as such either by his maturing reason or clarified and interpreted as such in therapy. Since they have no place in external reality, they dissolve when they become conscious and are understood. For Stephen, on the other hand, as for other seriously ill or damaged children, fantasy and reality coincide, the latter lending obvious backing to the former. Castration appears more feasible where limbs are actually attacked by illness and rendered useless; death for children with polio (especially before the Salk vaccine) was a frequent and dreaded occurrence which all children heard discussed. Even complete annihilation cannot seem impossible after the devastating experience of having one's whole life altered or shattered by catching an infection or by an accident. It is probably this addition of a terrifying reality to the usual frightening fantasy life of childhood which tips the scales for some children and presents them with a task which they cannot and do not want to solve.

TRIUMPH OF THE MIND OVER ILLNESS

CARL was a charming six-year-old when he contracted polio. It involved his entire body and he was completely paralyzed. Admitted first to a private room at University Hospitals, he immediately became the most admired and best-loved patient on his floor because of his cheerful attitude and courageous spirit. While his parents were distressed and terrified by the events, he only once showed fear of the respirator, which "might crush" him.

After three months he suddenly became withdrawn, was transferred to the children's ward for company, but remained solitary in spite of the adults' efforts to counteract his isolation. At Rainbow, where he was admitted a month later for convalescence, he appeared frail and sick. In spite of this, he remained cheerful and cooperative and began to relate to other children by being helpful and protective toward them. When his little neighbor wet his bed, he always comforted him: "Really, it does not matter, they don't mind it at all."

Carl's mother seldom visited him because she feared that her unhappiness might affect the child. His father, however, came every day and his entire conversation with Carl centered on sports. When he was warned that such discussions must be hard for the little boy, for whom there seemed no prospect at the time ever to participate in such activities, Mr. S. explained that he had great hopes in this respect for his son. He himself was considered the athletic type, and he thought it was of utmost importance to inspire the child in this way so that "he would work harder" to get well.

Carl still withdrew from the group whom he joined only when they had a party or cooked a meal; otherwise he preferred to play at bowling with his father.

Six months after the onset of illness, Carl started to attend school, worked extremely well, and, according to the teacher, was an interested and brilliant pupil. She commented especially on his courteous manners, which she considered outstanding for a child of his age. At the same time Carl was transferred from the polio unit to the Boys' Ward. He showed his pleasure openly because this had great meaning for him—a further step in his improvement. Again he received a great deal of attention from the children, their visitors, and the staff because of his charming and cheerful attitude.

Only gradually did it become obvious to us that Carl's personality achievements did not come easy to him and that he had to undergo internal struggles to cope with negative feelings such as jealousy of those who made a faster recovery, doubts about his own improvement, etc. The first indications of these were given by some stories he told of fights with Indians or robbers clashing with police. Nevertheless, even in these fantasies he usually remained the hero showing great strength and daring.

The next indication of Carl's conflict was seen in the appearance of some transitory symptoms none of which had a physical basis: fear of dizziness and of vomiting, and nosebleeds, all of which he used to avoid school or his physical therapy sessions.

When questioned about this by me, it emerged that his real fear was a different one: he was afraid that he might wet himself and, since he thought that children who did that had to go back into the respirator, he preferred not to be separated from his urinal. Actually, he brought his urinal with him when he came to discuss these matters with me, insisting that he "did not mind physical therapy," he "liked school," but only if he could be "prepared," i.e., have his urinal handy.

It seemed that Carl, who had never talked about his affliction, was using the question of wetting and its control to symbolize a whole turmoil of feelings: discontent with his own achievements (although at this time he could walk between the parallel bars, sit up very well, and use his hands and shoulders somewhat), disappointment when facing reality, fear of and longing for protection in the respirator. During this phase he could not bear to be praised for physical improvements, for example, for "walking well"; evidently they did not come up to his own standards.

The father's influence on the child was very apparent; the games and toys he bought and wanted Carl to play with were chosen for improving the muscles of his hands, rather than for fun. Carl asked me for assistance in learning to use these so as not to disappoint his father. He often became despondent when he realized that his handicap made these achievements a difficult task. The father readily agreed to accept guidance in choosing more adequate toys for Carl, but it was quite obvious that he could not really use advice in this respect. Nevertheless, I stressed with the father that Carl's scholastic achievements were outstanding and I thus hoped to transfer the ambitions he had for his son from sport to intellectual activities.

When the father told me about all the things he had provided at home in anticipation of Carl's return, he admitted very apologetically that he had also bought a bicycle: "I know he is not ready for it, but he came a long way and I promised it to him when he was better. I have to keep my promise—it might stimulate him to work hard to use it."

Carl was discharged on his seventh birthday, nine months after admission, at a time when he was able to walk approximately twelve steps in a corset. His shoulders, left arm and elbow were still weak. When told that he was about to return home, he dictated the following story which revealed to what a surprising degree this child too had experienced his illness as his own fault, and treatment and hospitalization as punishment and imprisonment from which one tries to escape.

THE STORY FOR A PUPPET SHOW

First there will be a big scream. And then a puppet will come out and announce the people.

Then a robber tries to get away from the bank. And the cops see him and shoot, but he gets away. But at night he comes back and shoots the cops, and the cops shoot him in the shoulder. Then he goes in his cabin which is his hide-out. Then the cops follow him and see him through the window and they surround the robber. But he shoots his way out. But then they had a fight and one of the cops shot him in the shoulder again. And then they took him to jail. And then he tried to get away, but he could not. And one of the prisoners said, "Why are you here?" And then he said, "I am here because I committed a crime." He stayed in prison for thirty years. And then they let him free. And again he had no money and he robbed all the places and the cops were looking for him again. They followed him and took him to prison again. And he stayed there for sixty-one years and when he got out he was no more of a bad guy and that is the way it all started and that is the way it all ended. That's all.

When two years later Carl was readmitted to Rainbow for treatment of scoliosis it was possible to assess the

Personality Development

progress he had made. At home he had walked well and even rode his bicycle. At Rainbow he now walked in his Riesser jacket, a top-heavy cast, and although he held on to things and people at first, Carl soon managed without canes or crutches. In his games with the other children he now played cops-and-robbers, whereas before he had merely dictated these stories. He liked to be jailkeeper and as such locked the "robbers" securely into the solarium. When he, in turn, played robber, he knew how to escape cunningly and later revealed his tricks with good humor and satisfaction. In short, he played like an active, normally aggressive little boy.

It is interesting to realize that the physical and medical evaluation could not explain how this child managed to walk so well with or without the cast because tests of muscle strength revealed quite insufficient power for such an accomplishment. With Carl it was evidently a case of "mind over matter." What had also to be taken into account was the father's denial of the facts, his unfaltering belief that everything was going to be all right again. Actually, it must have been the influence of the father's unrealistic attitude (and not my sensible advice) which contributed to Carl's amazingly successful recovery, the degree of which could not be explained in physical terms.

AN INSTITUTIONALIZED ILL CHILD

Larry, whom I met when he was eight, was a doubly deprived child. On the one hand, he was afflicted with tuberculosis of the hip, on the other hand he had missed family care most of his childhood, having been hospitalized in Rainbow from age three to age eleven. Under the conditions of treatment for his disease as they were at the time of his illness, he had had to undergo a great variety of procedures, including plaster casts, braces, Bradford frame, and traction. These had to be applied repeatedly when he relapsed after short-lived progress.

Larry's father, a case of arrested tuberculosis, had been in the hospital for long periods of time and blamed himself for having been the source of infection. Both parents had unfriendly relations with the hospital staff, a fact which did not remain without influence on Larry. They were demanding, difficult, and, finally, discouraged. Even when the policy at Rainbow changed from fortnightly to daily visiting, they did not take advantage of this and came only infrequently. The situation became even worse when a baby brother was born. The parents now had "a new Larry"; the mother was unable to come and the father had to refrain from visiting owing to a new flare-up of his own illness.

Like many other institutionalized children, Larry was completely unattached emotionally. Although he had received much kindness, care, and sympathy during his long years at Rainbow, there had also been during this period a complete change of administrative policy and many changes of staff. Interestingly enough he could not recall one single person or happening from this past, that is, before the time he met me. On the other hand, he talked about "going home," although his whole knowledge of being home since admission to the hospital consisted of three single week ends and one Christmas holiday at age six.

In his unhappy, sullen, and tempestuous state he was extremely difficult for the nursing staff to handle. Since he had intermittent rises of temperature, intermittent restrictions had to be imposed on him, which led to revolt against the nurses, anxiety attacks, and tantrums. Since the nurses were afraid to upset this delicate, ill child, he learned to use their reluctance to his advantage. He was disobedient and defiant. His favorite answers were: "So what, you cannot make me do it. You just try—just come near and I will kick you." Often he said simply: "I do not want to—that's all. Period."

Like many other unattached children, Larry took to stealing. His locker was often found to contain items which the other children claimed as their possessions. However, he insisted that he had found them or that they had been given to him as presents. He always denied vehemently having taken something—even if the other children had witnessed it. In defiance he told me, "I do not care if you don't believe me—nobody believes me—so what?" And after a pause he went on to say suddenly, "So what if I took it?" He lied if this was to his advantage. Like other children in his unhappy situation, he had never learned to set limits for himself for the sake of somebody he loved or for the sake of being loved.

With Larry all my efforts were directed toward establishing a meaningful relationship. Once I had become an important figure in his life, he revealed that the stealing was connected with his thoughts of home in two ways. He explained: "The others always have visitors who bring them things—well, you know I have no visitors, so I have no things either." It also emerged that he saved the stolen things to give as presents to his family; however, since the opportunity to do so hardly ever occurred, he usually ended up breaking them.

Going along with his fantasy that such gifts would buy the family's affection, I suggested that they would be better pleased if he made something by himself, a suggestion which turned his interest to handiwork for the first time and led to enjoyment of it. By next Christmas he had twenty-one presents ready; but even this was not enough for him and he proceeded to take, in addition, as many parcels as possible from under the Christmas tree, although they were gifts for the entire ward.

Larry never stole things from my office, although there was every opportunity to do so. He would examine toys which were there for the use of younger children and say: "What do you need that for? My baby brother would just love it."

I refused presents for the baby brother but was quite ready to give little gifts to him personally, not to be shared on the ward. These were cookies, pretzels, and the like, which had to be brought from my home, as a sign that I had thought of him. In the beginning he would start our sessions with the question: "Any goodies for me—from home?" Later, when he had become more sure of me, these tokens ceased to play an important part.

My explanations to him were simple ones: that it was not true that he did not care about anybody or anything; how much he wanted to be liked; that one could not buy affection; that it was not enough to say to me "I like you all right," that he would also have to please me; that I did not like to hear that he had kicked another child, or been angry when told to go to bed, etc.

My next step was to help him transfer his newly found affections to a particular nurse with whom he gradually developed an extremely good relationship. "I am her pet and I want to be her pet." While he still had many altercations with the other staff members, he tried to be at his best behavior when she cared for him, until he learned to please her by being good in her absence as well. Once, when punished and taken out of the group while she was away, he wrote her a pathetic little letter: "I know you don't like me now, but I still love you." Gradually his temper tantrums diminished and his stealing ceased. He had passed through a phase of development which other children accomplish in their earliest years under the affectionate guidance of their parents.

Larry's situation took a definite turn for the better when the surgeon decided to excise a lesion of his hip and held out hope to the parents that, following this, he would be ready to go home. It was my difficult task to prepare him rather hurriedly for this operation. At first Larry was adamant when I introduced the plan of surgery to him. This had the flavor of an emergency and therefore aroused even more fear and anxieties in him.

"Oh no. I won't have any part of it," he kept on saying and he sounded quite determined. "I will not have it. Period. Not me. Nobody can make me go. Not me. Oh no, sir. My parents would not want me to have it, that I am sure."

I explained, "Yes, they think it would be better for you to have this operation because then you would not have these flare-ups of fever and pain. They think it would be better because you could go home sooner."

"I will go home soon, but no operation. No, thank you. Remember John? He had a stiff hip. Who wants a stiff hip? I could never play football with a stiff hip."

Suddenly Larry started to cry, realizing that he never had played football, nor did it seem possible that he ever would with a hip condition that caused so many setbacks throughout the years.

"You have another leg to kick the ball—but you have to

be well to be on the field. You could learn to run fast enough, even with a stiff hip," I told him.

Finally, Larry gave in, helped toward acquiescence by his confidence in the nurse and me and by the hope of returning "home."

The final outcome was a happy one. After successful surgery, he was accepted into his family and settled down. His physical condition remained satisfactory. He became a good student at school and was even reported to be efficient on the football field.

13

Arthritic and Asthmatic Patients: Involvement with the Mother

In contrast to most other patients who during prolonged hospitalization turned to the staff for relief and comfort, children with arthritis and asthma hardly ever shifted their allegiance away from their mothers. The interplay with the mother seemed to have a massive beneficial or pernicious influence on the course of illness.

ARTHRITIC CHILDREN

While all ill children feel more secure in the presence of their mothers, those afflicted with arthritis also seem to expect their mothers to relieve the pain, which in their case is excruciating and on which they concentrate. It was not unusual for our arthritic children to suffer an attack of acute pain merely because the mother's planned visit was canceled. It was also not unusual for the mothers under our observation to respond to their child's expectation with helplessness and guilt feelings, to which the children in their turn reacted.

ANN, aged eight, was typical in this respect. She was quiet, obedient, withdrawn into herself. To change the wedges in her cast, the plaster had to be cut every week, a simple procedure to which the child nevertheless reacted with vehement outbursts of fear. However, when, to prevent the accompanying relapses, her mother was allowed to be present, Ann showed no fear at all and instead made fun of her own cowardice.

Even in periods when she had no pain, Ann needed her mother to make decisions for her. Without that, she felt lost and forlorn, and rather than decide for herself, broke into tears, which in their turn brought on attacks of pain.

When Ann was at home, the mother became responsible for the child's rather painful exercises—a task which the mother found especially difficult. It did not fit into the relationship built up between them that she should inflict pain rather than remove it. "I never know what to do. I know she is in pain, then I worry and her pain gets worse." With Ann, as with others, we were familiar with a typical vicious circle: pain causing withdrawal and depression, and the depressed mood in turn intensifying pain. Sometimes this circle could be broken and the child comforted and cheered up; but usually this role was reserved for the mother alone.

MAY was separated from her mother when she was two years old and placed with a good foster mother. At age three she developed rheumatoid arthritis and in the year that followed she was hospitalized at Rainbow twice, the second time in poor condition, very ill, emaciated, her limbs deformed, her joints badly swollen. She remained motionless, in pain, and apathetic, with no interest in any friendliness shown her.

Like Ann, she was unable to make decisions and express preferences. Even when she was asked whether she would rather sit up or lie down, she would become unhappy and cry, feeling protected only when told what to do. As she explained later: "I was just scared of people when they asked me. They knew anyway what I wanted." She lost weight continuously since she refused almost everything that was offered or, at best, accepted only minute quantities of food.

When May was referred to me, I found it very difficult to open up communication with her. In her extreme withdrawal she did not talk and showed no interest in toys. At first, I had to be content with the fact that she tolerated my visits and, gradually, seemed pleased by the regularity with which I appeared. Cautiously, to draw some of her interest away from herself, I introduced two tiny goldfish which she consented to watch and—since living creatures have to eat—to feed with my help.

As a next step, I made some paper dolls, as far as possible in her own image, and some paper furniture, weightless enough for her fingers to handle. These dolls also wanted to eat, and I succeeded in getting May to order their food from me, which I drew: hamburgers, wieners, sauerkraut and pickles, i.e., whatever she had been accustomed to before her illness, the dolls' favorite dish being, surprisingly enough, mustard sandwiches. It was a great victory when, finally, she could be induced to taste the dolls' fantasy lunch in reality and, in this way, become able to regain some pleasure in and tolerance for nourishment.

In striking contrast to May's alarming difficulties at this time, six months later things took a turn for the better when May's own mother visited her. The child was overjoyed, began to play with a little record player which the mother had brought, and learned to handle it herself in spite of stiff and swollen fingers. At the same time all the presents brought by the foster mother were ignored and the woman herself was treated with hostility until she ceased coming. May talked only of going home to her own mother. "My mummy will see to it that I never again get sick."

From then onward, May's physical condition went up and down, depending on the mother's interest in her. When the mother made the necessary adjustments to provide a suitable home for the child, May walked well on crutches. When the stress at home became too great, May deteriorated and had to return to Rainbow. To go home again, she learned to walk without crutches, an achievement which elated her. When for three years the mother surpassed all our expectations in caring for the child, May did extremely well physically and did well in school. When the home broke up again, she became quite ill and needed intensive medical care.

At one time, in the hospital, she retold the story of "Rapunzel," revealing in it her own thoughts and anxieties:

> Once upon a time there was a girl and her name was Mary. She lived in a big castle. She was a princess. She was pretty. She had long hair. She had a real long dress made of white silk. She liked to look out of the window all day long. But

she could not do that because the witch would get her. The witch wanted the princess to stay with her. The Mummy and Daddy did not want the princess to be with the witch, but they *had* to because the witch would get them. When the princess was a tiny baby, when she was born, the witch saw the man. And then he took a lettuce. The witch said, "When your baby is born you must give it to me." And the man said "O.K.," and he did. Now the man was a king. And the witch came to take the baby, they did not want to, but they *had* to. Then the princess was sad with the witch and said she wanted to go home because the witch looked funny and mean. The princess cried and cried all day. Then she saw the prince and he made a ladder for her and it took a real long time. Before the prince went into the army he showed the girl the way and she sneaked away. And her Mummy said, "Who is she?" and her Daddy said, "Who is that?" And she said, "That's *Mary*." And they said, "Oh, I know her."

JOYCE[1] was an arthritic child, largely deprived of her mother's care, much as she would have needed it in her illness, a fact which had serious effects on her personality development. She developed rheumatoid arthritis at the age of five and from five to fifteen spent part of every year at Rainbow. The mother was poor, responsible for six children, two of whom were severely handicapped. The one time in her life when Joyce was in sole possession of the mother, her siblings being with the grandmother, she was free of pain.

[1] See also Chapter 9.

Like other children who are deprived of their mother's care when the need for it is at its height, Joyce reacted by caring for herself, i.e., by becoming self-centered and hypochondriacal, looking after herself and her own body as if mothering herself. When at the age of nine she improved miraculously with the help of cortisone therapy, instead of enjoying it to the full, she persisted in her hypochondriacal attitude, was constantly concerned about herself, and kept on asking when her uptime was over. She would look unhappily at her food: "Sure, I love chili, but does it have enough protein for me?"

For her body's sake she did not mind returning to Rainbow periodically, but she warded off contacts, wanted to be left alone, and was concerned exclusively with her condition, her appearance, her hair, her own person, her likes and dislikes. This attitude extended to her medical treatments where she wanted to decide herself what should be done, and she could not be persuaded by the nurses or therapist to follow the doctor's orders if she herself had ruled against them.

That Joyce's excessive independence was no more than a defense, a desperate attempt to mother herself in the absence of being mothered, was shown at other times when it broke down completely. Then, usually when readmittance to the hospital became necessary on medical grounds, she suddenly let herself go, became unkempt and disheveled, i.e., presented herself as much in need of care as the lost and forlorn waif she really felt she was.

ASTHMATIC CHILDREN

It is well known that unrealistic distortions of the mother-child interaction also play their part in childhood asthma. While these distortions can be fully understood only in analytic treatment, observations in the hospital permitted identification of at least a few facts and recurring patterns.

An unusually bizarre case was that of Mrs. M. and her child—bizarre, that is, if viewed in terms of the mother's behavior. This young woman had herself suffered from asthma and had been told by a physician that her own condition had predisposed the child to the disease. Nevertheless she clung to the belief that unusual events during her pregnancy had caused the child's illness. She felt that she herself had been cured by a "miracle," which occurred while she, as a side-show lady, found that she could tolerate massive electric currents being sent through her body. She expected a similar miracle to happen to her child and had waited patiently for it for five years, during which she had neglected to seek medical treatment for the girl. While we tried to disentangle and understand her irrational attitude, it became clear to her that, in fact, she had condemned herself to the hardship and worry caused by her child's attacks in retribution for the suffering which she as a child, owing to her asthma, had inflicted on her own mother.

Judy, aged eight, presented another example of the complex mother-child relationship of asthmatic children.

With asthma beginning at eleven months, Judy had experienced twenty-two emergency admissions to hospitals prior to coming to Rainbow. On arrival, she looked ill, emaciated, old, and shriveled, and was moaning loudly during an attack. She presented a completely different picture on the next day when she was free from wheezing.

The history given by Judy's mother included sudden weaning at eleven months for hospitalization, and very early toilet training already completed at that age. The mother also admitted that she had always had a very special relationship to this child, different from that to her first-born; she carried the baby all the time, even while doing housework and cooking; she slept in the same bed with her—all against her husband's remonstrations. When the child was in school, she had often "simply felt" that she had to call the school, only to be told that Judy had "just had an attack." (While Judy was in the hospital the mother, in addition to visiting daily, telephoned every morning at seven o'clock for information about attacks.) Judy had always had fewer attacks when her father had looked after her while her mother was at work.

Judy was proud of her hospitalizations: "They give you a shot and you right away feel better. I got three shots a day and the other children only got one. . . . I was much longer in the oxygen tent. . . . Did you see my chart, it is thicker than a telephone directory," etc.

There was evidence that the mother's early weaning and toilet training had left their mark on Judy. In attacks she got relief from the inhaler, but used it as a pacifier, even an empty one serving the purpose. Her ambivalence showed in the many broken inhalers, smashed carelessly, which on the other hand had to be replaced hurriedly to avoid despair. Medication given orally brought immediate relief, long before it could have had a pharmacological effect. Suppositories acted similarly, making her "feel good" instantaneously, even when they were—experimentally—applied plain, without medication. In the same oral-anal context she resisted procedures for removal of mucus to ease breathing.

ARTHRITIC AND ASTHMATIC CHILDREN   125

There was no doubt in anybody's mind that for Judy her debilitating illness provided the means of clinging to a very infantile level of relationship with her mother. Her attitude to inhaler, suppositories, and swallowing of mucus represented the reverse of her early compliance with toilet training and weaning which had taken place in the overheated, overpossessive relationship of this mother with her child.

MARION's case confirmed that swallowing of mucus is characteristic of many asthmatic children.[2] According to Marion's mother, the child could not be taught to blow her nose; she simply swallowed her mucus during crying spells, thereby causing coughing and wheezing. Marion's personality structure bore out the anal nature of this symptom. She hoarded and collected; hardly playing with her many toys, she wanted more and more, duplicating those she had. She asked for things worthless to others, boxes, ribbons, string, paper, saving it all carefully. She avoided paint, clay, paste, etc., intent on keeping clean. Obviously, while conforming in every other way to the mother's ideal of a clean child, her symptom provided the only means of being "dirty." She saved her phlegm as she saved the small items which she wished to have "for keeps."

Since Marion continually had attacks at home, she was never thwarted and she used her power. In the hospital, when I could not supply the drink she fancied, she fell into despair, calling, "Mummy—Mummy—Mummy," crying, swallowing tears and mucus, coughing, emulating what she did at home—but, interestingly, she did *not* wheeze. After stopping, she accepted what I had to offer,

[2] For additional material concerning Marion, see Chapter 7.

asking: "Why do I always have to call my mummy?" In her case as well, the asthmatic reaction seemed tied to the mother's presence.

During five months at Rainbow Marion had only one slight episode of wheezing which occurred upon her return from a week end at home.

It is often thought that the improvements asthmatic children show in the hospital are due to dust-free surroundings, a more suitable heating system, etc. However, Rainbow was not as dust-free as Judy's and Marion's homes, which had been equipped especially in this respect. Nor did the dust-free or smoke-free atmosphere bring improvement in the case of Sally.

SALLY, after the initial acute episode, was free of attacks during her stay at Rainbow. However, whenever she returned from week-end visits at home, she was so sick that she needed most of the following week to recuperate. Her mother, convinced that the heating system in their house was responsible, took rooms in a motel to give her "a good enjoyable week end." However, this did not prevent the set pattern from recurring and Sally (then about nine years old) was not spared the most severe attacks.

Sally told about her attacks at home which occurred mostly at night after her father returned from work. "I know it's all in my lungs, but when I see that coat—I always think it is a monster. My father always puts it there for me to see and get used to. I know it's only an old coat, but when I look at it, it's 'Frankenstein!' He is a monster and comes at night and sits on people's chests and he squeezes their neck until they cannot breathe and their heads fall off."

Although most physicians today take it for granted that asthma is not a purely physical but a psychosomatic disease, the exact details of the pathogenic interplay between mind and body still await elucidation. On the mental side, shortcomings and dissatisfactions in the early mother-child relationship; excessive anxiety, overindulgence or overprotectiveness on the part of the mother; an oral disposition and the fact of certain archaic fantasies on the part of the child have all been cited as causative factors. Anxieties, aggressions, and emotional upsets obviously serve to aggravate the patient's condition.

What we could observe in the hospital, from the behavioral side, was the way in which the asthmatic child watched and expected his breathing to become more and more laborious, how his anxiety mounted parallel with the acute discomfort, to become overwhelming during the attack. It seemed understandable enough that at the height of this anxiety the children turned for support to their own mothers and not to us. Furthermore, the children knew that their slightest wheezing in the presence of the mother would arouse the same anxiety in her that they themselves felt. This common reaction intensified the already excessive bond between mother and child in all our cases.

On the other hand, it is characteristic of asthma that, once established, it is not relieved but aggravated by the mother's presence. Asthmatic children regularly improve when taken out of their environment. At Rainbow it was often demonstrated medically that separation had been physically beneficial, aiding treatment, clearing the lung fields, etc.

Usually the improvements brought about by hospitalization, remarkable as they were in some instances, were not maintained after the child returned home. In view of the deep-seated nature of psychosomatic disturbances this could hardly be otherwise. However, the mere fact that separation had resulted in improvement was often sufficient to encourage the parents to consider either long-term placement or analytic treatment for their child.

14

Return Home

While admission techniques such as those developed at Rainbow Hospital have in many instances been successful in easing the child's transition from normal life to a restricted hospital existence, less attention has been paid to the other end of the hospital experience: to what happens when the child leaves the hospital and returns to his community. Where our own patients are concerned, we lack any systematic or comprehensive follow-ups of their adjustments. All we possess so far is chance information about some and a whole host of questions waiting to be answered.

There is no doubt that in all our patients' minds "going home" existed as a wholly pleasurable fantasy, endowed with magic expectations to which they clung. Nevertheless, in many instances the distance between this imaginary picture and its realization was considerable.

For some children hospital life undoubtedly made

fewer demands on their abilities than home life; the physical surroundings were better suited to their limited capacities to move about or go outdoors independently; they had made valuable contacts and been provided with entertaining and educational activities. Even the routine itself often gave a feeling of security.

When DANNY, aged eight, returned home he could not understand why his breakfast was not served at 8:15, his lunch at 11:30, and his afternoon nap began punctually. He had become accustomed to taking his medication at set times and to making ready for physical therapy at others, and he missed this. Although he was happy that his physical improvement permitted him to go home, Danny was concerned that he would get worse again if he was not taken care of as in the hospital.

While some children showed no ambivalent feelings when going home and gladly left their friends and the hospital to become engrossed in new experiences, others were openly reluctant or even acted out their unwillingness to leave by having falls or injuries which prolonged their stay. With them, evidently, their mental readiness for resuming normal life was not keeping pace with physical recovery.

We know little, so far, about the long-term aftereffects of chronic illness on personality development. That the degree of residual physical impairment does not in itself determine success or failure of adaptation is evidenced by experience. Robert, deaf and blind, found a successful place in life after discharge; Gene, with no more than a slight limp, was possessed by the desire to compensate for this by driving cars at a furious speed, until he lost his life in a driving accident. Braces, casts, or even existence in a wheel chair were often tolerated more easily than minor impairments which make competition with the healthy world a possibility.

On the other hand, of course, adaptation could be seen to depend on the home atmosphere to which the child returned. Some parents seemed unable themselves to come to terms with the child's handicap or not to trust themselves sufficiently to assume responsibility for aftercare. For the professionally untaught the handling of even a partially disabled child presents many difficulties, and in this realm nurses, physical therapist, and I could be of decisive help.

In observing from a distance the further development of discharged patients, we were impressed by the mothers' decisive role in guiding the children toward satisfactory adjustment to the home environment and toward integrating and overcoming the shocks of hospital experience.

An example of this was NANCY who, after surgery of the spine and a long convalescence, had readjusted to life with the assistance of an unusually understanding mother —to the extent that Nancy was now ready to give similar help to others. At the age of thirteen she wrote the following letter to Jackie, a boy of five, who was being prepared for the same operation:[1]

> Dear Jackie,
> My name is Nancy M. and I had the same kind of operation that you are going to have, so I

[1] For further attempts to prepare Jackie, see Chapter 7.

thought maybe you would like to know a little about it.

First of all, I have to admit I was rather afraid at first, but you need not worry about that because the nurse will give you a certain medicine that will help you relax and get unafraid.

When the operation is over it will hurt some, but right away the nurse will give you some medicine for that too. Then for about four or five days you will probably want to rest a lot and by the end of this time you will begin to feel much better.

When the doctor puts you in your body cast it may be a little uncomfortable for you at first, for about a week, but then you get pretty well settled to it. You will be able to do almost everything except walk or sit up. So when you are all finished I think you will be very glad you went through with it. I know I am. In fact, I am walking now and feeling just fine with my walking cast. I am home now and will miss seeing you.

Then too you can look forward to coming to Rainbow Hospital and staying for a while. I think you will like it much better than B & C or whatever hospital where you will have the operation. There is much more to do at Rainbow than there is at any other hospital and I think you will enjoy it very much.

So I wish you all the luck in the world and again I say I think you will be very glad you went through with it all.

Lots of luck,
Nancy

Part III

CONCLUSION

15

Conclusion

When assessing the practical value of the material presented in the preceding pages, a number of considerations have to be taken into account, such as the following:

SEVERE, CHRONIC VERSUS MINOR, ACUTE ILLNESS

It is a characteristic of this book that the author's observations are derived from work with children whose lives were disrupted by the most dangerous and crippling bodily afflictions. Nevertheless it seems to us erroneous to conclude that this diminishes its relevance for those parents, nurses or physicians who deal habitually with the more benign and transitory forms of children's diseases. The differences to be noted in the patients' reactions to the two types of illness are matters of degree and quantity rather than basic differences in quality; more important still, they concern external physical realities rather than the internal psychic realities of the child, with all the discrepancies which exist between the former and the latter.

So far as *surgery* is concerned, for example, any interference with the child's body, whether major or minor, is likely to arouse his fantasies and fears with regard to being attacked, mutilated, deprived of a valuable part of his own self. It makes surprisingly little difference whether the intervention is as serious as in the cases of Linda (Chapter 7) or Jackie (Chapter 7), or as insignificant as with Marion (Chapter 7). Whatever has been seen in one of the children described above is also present in the usual cases of tonsillectomy, adenoidectomy or hernia repair, occasions which are regarded by many of the children concerned with no less dread than Carl regarded being placed in the respirator (Chapter 11) or with which Henry (Chapter 8) and Larry (Chapter 12) met their dangerous operations.

On the other hand, the differences between major and minor, serious and negligible, which are insufficiently reacted to by the child patient himself, loom very large in the minds of the medical and nursing staff, who are used to an objective and wholly realistic appraisal of events. Our attempts to reveal the children's intimate reactions may be met with incredulity by the adults in question so long as they concern procedures which are harmless and insignificant to their eyes, as are impending visits to the dentist, injections, inoculations, or completely noninjurious events such

CONCLUSION 137

as sun-ray treatments. What blocks understanding here is the normal adult's unfamiliarity with the child's subjective, irrational, emotional approach. Adult understanding comes more readily where psychic reality and external reality coincide and the child's fears are concerned with unquestionably serious situations which cannot fail to evoke anybody's concern and sympathy; on the other hand, once the child's helpless terror has been brought home to the environment on these occasions, it is easier to establish the fact that, so far as fantasies, anxieties, and affects are concerned, the piercing of a boil, the taking of a blood sample, or the extraction of a tooth may loom as large as the actual removal of an eye or the amputation of a limb. What needs to be understood is the fact that in both instances, whether objectively justified or not, the patient's emotions are very real and the child is in need of help. That in this book's exposition the reader is invited to follow a path of understanding which leads from the major to the minor events may well have its advantages over the usual course which goes in the opposite direction.

As regards the child's conception of *illness as punishment*, there is a similar lack of difference between severe illness and its lighter forms. Any intercurrent infection, caught inadvertently, is understood by many children as the consequence of naughtiness and revives the memory of things eaten, warm clothing and rubbers discarded or fought against, puddles walked into, etc., in the face of parental prohibition. What weighs heavily on the child in these instances is neither the actual act of disobedience, nor its alleged bodily consequence as such, but their symbolic value, namely, what appears to the child as a confirmation of the belief that wrongdoing, however secretly performed, is open to punishment, and that other, still undetected misdeeds, whether actually carried out or merely contemplated in fantasy, will likewise be followed by retribution of some kind. This idea intensifies all the fears which in any case accompany childhood development, and it arouses intolerable pangs of conscience irrespective of whether fate metes out the supposed "punishment" in the form of rheumatic illnesses, as with Ernest (Chapter 10) or Ruth (Chapter 10), or in the milder form of common colds, sore throats, upsets of the stomach and digestive tract, etc.

Even with respect to the *duration of illness*, the enormous difference between the chronic and acute states is significant for the adult environment rather than for the children themselves, especially for the younger ones. This of course does not mean that a year (or more) of hospitalization or bodily incapacity seems short to any child; even the shortest terms of being confined, of being in the hospital, on a diet, under motor restriction, etc., seem intolerably long or even eternal to all children, whether they last twenty-four hours, three days, a week or a fortnight. The operative factor here is that the sense of time functions differently in earlier than in later ages. Adults behave objectively about time; i.e., they measure it with the help of clock and calendar, and this reality-adapted attitude gives way only occasionally, when time "passes incredibly quickly" with some pleasurable occupation; or when it "drags on," "hangs heavy on their hands," appears "interminable" when they are bored, or in pain, or anxiously awaiting some event. In the very young, however, these latter subjective appraisals of time are the order of the day—in fact, are the only attitude to time of which they are capable. Not only are calendar and clock still beyond their intellectual grasp; it is of greater importance that their measuring of time is carried out not by their ego, i.e., the sensible and rational part of their personalities, but by the strength and urgency of their wishes which turn all periods of time into waiting times, namely, waiting for gratification of their impulses. What young children, especially those of the toddler age, accomplish least of all is postponement of wish fulfillment, whether the wish is a crudely instinctual one or merely a wish for comfort, company, entertainment, activity, motor outlet, relief from discomfort, pain or anxiety. Consequently, all periods of illness are painfully long for the child, whatever their objective length. Here too, understanding is easier for the adults if they acquire their insights from contact with the chronic rather than the acute illnesses. In cases of the first kind the child's despair about the duration of his incapacity is readily grasped and shared by parents and hospital staff, whereas his fretting and impatience in the case of short, acute spells is dismissed more easily as "unreasonable" and, consequently, met with little sympathy or with facile promises that discomfort or deprivation will "soon be over," "not last long," "only take a minute," i.e., with reassurances which are out of harmony with the child's inner experience and therefore fail to be effective in allaying his anxieties.

Finally, so far as the *study of children's reactions to illness* is concerned in general, there are obvious advantages offered by a hospital setting such as Rainbow's. In the usual quick turnover of a general pediatric ward, there is little for the observer to see apart from the immediate impact on the children of separation from home, admission to unfamiliar surroundings, with the consequent reactions of shock, or anxiety, or protest, or withdrawal, etc., often intermixed and overlaid with attitudes of apparent indifference, compliance, and acceptance. The acutely ill patient, in contrast to the chronic one, has no time to proceed beyond the distress of the unrelated newcomer, to transfer confidence and dependence onto the hospital staff, and to change thereby from a shadowy figure to a distinct individual, revealing the doubts, conflicts, difficulties, and fantasies about his illness which we have described above. On the other hand, it is precisely this intimate, personal knowledge of the child on which help, support, and reassurance for him can be based; and it is easier to apply to the acutely ill patients what has been learned in the orthopedic, tuberculosis or poliomyelitis hospitals than to gather the necessary insights during the hurried contacts with the shifting population of an ear, nose, and throat ward.

INTERACTION BETWEEN MIND AND BODY

If, as the authors hope, the descriptions given in this book are accepted as valid, it may be permitted to extract from them some conclusions as to the normal interactions between mind and body in the early ages.

In our time, when the *psychosomatic* basis of many illnesses is in the process of being accepted by the medical profession, it seems hardly necessary to present additional examples of "mind over matter" or to stress the importance of emotional factors in such illnesses as asthma, certain heart conditions, etc. It is also a well-known fact that the younger the child, the closer is normally the connection between mind and body, because, in the relative absence of mental outlets through thinking, reasoning, and speech, the emotions are discharged through physical channels via skin eruptions, upsets in the feeding and sleeping rhythm, the digestive tract, etc. Therefore, what we tried to illustrate in the preceding chapters is no more than the experience that, even in the severe illnesses of our organic patients, attitudes and emotions such as hope, despair, compliance, fear, guilt, etc., played a part, precipitating the onset of the disease or contributing to it, delaying recovery or speeding it up, as with Elizabeth (Chapter 10), and occasionally even determining the final outcome in a positive or negative direction (see Stephen, Chapter 12, and Carl, Chapter 11).

Compared with the attention paid to psychosomatic factors, the *impact of physical happenings on the mind* and on personality formation constitutes a neglected chapter; we have tried, accordingly, to document it amply in the preceding pages.

The medical and nursing personnel must inevitably be guided in their actions by the needs which arise during the various physical crises or the exigencies of pre- and postoperative situations. This, nevertheless, does not alter the fact that every single happening during illness, as well as every single action performed during its course and for its sake, beneficial as it may be in the physical sense, also has its potential adverse repercussions on the child's mind. The following are merely some representative examples of these:

1. The mere incidence of pain and discomfort, especially in early infancy, upsets the delicate *balance between pleasure and unpleasure,* which lies at the basis of mental development and determines the infant's positive or negative attitude to life. We know now that the newborn's earliest concept of himself is located in the kernel of pleasurable sensations connected with the physical experiences of feeding, satiation, body comfort, etc. The infant "loves" all these pleasures and shrinks from all experiences of pain and discomfort, which have a retarding and disrupting effect on his ego growth. For this reason, painful illnesses at the beginning of life, as well as painful medical procedures, are justifiably dreaded in the interest of mental development.

2. Another potential interference with the progressive personality development of the older child is the

situation of *"being nursed,"* and this quite apart from and often in striking contrast to his physical need for the nurse's help. Adult patients who, while healthy, feel certain of their independence in body matters can during physical illness permit themselves to return temporarily to the state of a helpless infant whose body is under other people's care and jurisdiction. It is impossible for children to accept nursing in the same spirit. For them, to have attained a measure of physical independence from the adult world and to have personal control over their own bodies are great developmental achievements which they prize highly and are reluctant to renounce. They may show this by obstructive and uncooperative behavior as a defense against the regressive move which the situation demands from them (Stephen, Chapter 12); or they may feel unable to keep up their more mature status and slip back entirely into passive compliance, allowing themselves to be handled without resistance (Keith, Chapter 8; Harriet, Chapter 11). Both reactions are unwelcome and unhelpful, from the practical point of view of dealing with the ill body as well as from the aspect of smooth, progressive mental development.[1]

3. It is not difficult to understand that nursing and medical staff feel reluctant if they are asked to take into account the meaning which their handling has for the child, i.e., of the fantastic interpretations and

[1] Adult men who ward off latent passive-feminine tendencies in their personality structure are often notoriously bad patients. Like the children, they put up a fight against the passive experience of being nursed.

transformations which their practical actions undergo in the child's mind. Not every child is objective enough to praise the nurse as a "corker," because she pursues her course of action dutifully, regardless of his protests (see Dave, Chapter 11). Most children are, instead, in the grip of the fears and fantasies which are touched on and reinforced by the physical experience. Thus, the taking of a blood sample is translated into an attack by hostile forces (Marion, Chapter 7). Operations are registered in the mind as interference with the intactness of the body and experienced according to age and level of development as annihilation, mutilation, or castration.

Hospitalization or isolation because of infection gives substance to ever-present fears of being rejected and of being unworthy. Diets are reacted to as deprivations and are experienced as especially intolerable when there is a strong fixation to the oral infantile phase, during which food and love are equated by the child. Medical investigations are feared by many children because they are "examinations" in the true sense of the word, i.e., inspections of the body which may reveal damage self-inflicted through masturbation, etc. (Gene, Chapter 8). Circumcision, if performed after infancy, is invariably interpreted as punishment. Medical interferences with the body openings (such as enemas, ear sprays) are reacted to as if they were acts of seduction. Painful procedures of all kinds are apt to arouse and make manifest in many children their latent masochistic tendencies (see Donna, Chapters 6 and 8).

The point is frequently made that it would add to the heavy burden carried by the hospital staff if emotional implications were taken seriously by them, alongside the physical ones with which they are concerned. Whether this would in fact be the case is still an open question. As matters stand at present, no greater gulf can be imagined than that existing between the practical, factual, and realistic approach of most medical and nursing personnel on the pediatric wards and the unrealistic, affective response of their patients—a gulf which in many instances precludes cooperation and the building up of positive relationships, and causes as much exasperation on one side as it causes distress and unhappiness on the other. As pointed out in the introduction, it is as much the task of the "hospital therapist" to introduce the staff to the intricacies of the child patient's mental and emotional functioning as it is her task to guide the children toward a clearer grasp of the physical and medical necessities. In our opinion, such advances toward mutual understanding do not add complications to the situation. On the contrary, they can serve only to ease the present strain on both parties, to clear the atmosphere, and thereby to improve the conditions which are favorable for the process of recovery.

THE TECHNIQUE OF "MENTAL FIRST AID" IN THE CHILDREN'S HOSPITAL

After reading what we have to offer, people may complain that our book contains no clear-cut guidance on two important topics: (1) how to gain access to those intimacies of the child patient on the knowledge of which help for him has to be based; (2) and how to determine what form of help should be offered in the various instances. Although procedures are described with regard to many individual cases, no clues are given why they were selected; whether it is reasoning or intuition by which the hospital therapist was prompted to spin out preparation for surgery with Harriet (Chapter 7) while hastening it with Marion (Chapter 7); to respect Donna's defensive denial (Chapter 11) while working to replace it with Betty (Chapter 11) by a more realistic attitude; to reassure some children while simply allowing Ruby's (Chapter 7) grief to run its course.

All we can offer in our defense is that the omission of such answers is neither accidental nor unintentional. In spite of the urgent need for an acceptable and accepted technique of "mental first aid" in the hospital, so far no such technique is in existence. Even though attempts in this direction are being undertaken in various places,[2] none of them have gone far enough, or been proved valid enough, to be published, taught, and generally recommended. Up to now, this type of work is in the experimental stage, and it is left to the discretion of each pioneering worker to open up the path of communication with the child patients and to choose appropriate remedies for the internal difficulties and complexities which are encountered. That such a method is one of trial and error is unavoidable;

[2] Among others, in the Kinderkliniek Academisch Ziekenhuis in Leiden, Holland under Prof. N. G. M. Veeneklaas.

on the whole this seems preferable to the authors than to advocate ready-made solutions before their validity has been tested sufficiently and their worth been proved.

With regard to the actual procedures adopted for the cases described above, all that can be said of them is that, according to the need of the moment, they were borrowed from a number of other fields and adapted *ad hoc* to the given conditions of the hospital environment, the fields being those of child rearing, education, play therapy, child guidance, and child analysis. As mentioned before, the understanding of the facts observed was based throughout on the psychoanalytic theory of child development which implies that children, while emotionally dependent on their parents, are personalities in their own right with their own underworld of instincts and desires; their own consciences and demands on themselves; and their own rational ego trying to keep the balance between impulse and ideals and with it between the pressures from the inner and the outer world. While this task of achieving a relative inner balance is not an easy one for any child, it is taken for granted here that it becomes immeasurably more difficult when anxieties, frustrations, and deprivations due to illness are added to it.

So far as establishing actual contact with the child's inner world is concerned, this does not seem to us to present insuperable difficulties. This type of communication is based on the fact that children have a natural need and wish to confide and share their feelings. In the absence of the parents they transfer this wish to a substitute figure if given the time, the opportunity, and the privacy to do so, the last named probably being the most difficult to achieve under conditions of the ward. In the presence of the parents, it is the latter's positive relations to the hospital which enable the child to displace his confidence and communicate freely without experiencing a conflict of loyalty. Only where the child himself is oblivious of the true cause of his distress does this natural approach need reinforcement from the recognized techniques of how to undo inner defenses and unravel the processes of the unconscious mind.

To apply these remarks in greater detail to our cases:

There are simple, human situations where the hospital therapist is called upon merely to assume the mother's basic role of *giving comfort*. As in the case of Ruby (Chapter 7), this usually happens when the mother herself is too distressed and shaken by the event to perform her task.

Likewise, in the cases of Linda, Harriet, Jane, and Jackie (all described in Chapter 7), the hospital therapist usurped a task which normally falls within the province of an understanding mother. In fact, no young child is able to weather the ups and downs of external reality without being swamped by fear, guilt, and anxiety-arousing fantasies. To keep up a reality-adapted attitude he has to lean heavily on the mature reason of the mother, whose role it is to clarify the issues and to remove over and over again the misunderstandings derived from his emotional irrationality and his primitive defensive ways of coping with events, reversing affects to the contrary ones, denying facts and necessities, etc. Where, for some reason such as absence, lack of understanding, lack of sympathy, the mother herself fails the child in this respect, the role of *"auxiliary ego"* can be taken over profitably by the hospital therapist.

In Marion's case (Chapter 7), the hospital therapist acted as *educators* do, namely, on the intuition that an authoritative decision by the adult can be helpful in putting an end to situations where the child's complaints and hesitations serve ulterior motives such as attention seeking, provocation, masochism. When intuition is right, the intervention acts as a relief for the child, as it did for Marion. On the other hand, there are no real safeguards against guessing wrong or against basing the decision not on the child's need but on the adult's exasperation with the child's unreasonable attitude.

With May's food refusal (Chapter 13) and Jane's preparation for surgery (Chapter 7) the method used was that of *play therapy*, i.e., inducing the child to displace the area of anxiety or conflict to the dolls and using the dolls to play out solutions which are then secondarily applied to the child herself.

In the cases of Ronnie (Chapter 5) and Larry (Chapter 12) success was achieved by means of *"corrective experience,"* a method of therapy which usually is effective only with the very young. To make up for the mother's strict handling (with Ronnie) or the mother's neglect (with Larry), the therapist, and the nurses under her direction, assumed the role of permissive and caring mother figures in relation to whom the child was able to lessen conflicts and take forward steps in development—an achievement which the child had been unable to accomplish in relation to the real mother.

With Ernest, Cindy, and Ruth (all three described in Chapter 10) the procedure resembled that in the usual child *guidance treatment* where, after the child's confidence has been won, guilt feelings and masturbation conflicts are verbalized, discussed, and relieved. While these conflicts lay near the surface of the mind, with no real obstacle blocking these children's awareness of the problem, the situation was different in the case of Elizabeth (Chapter 10). With her, the connections had to be pursued patiently from the subject of the bad, seducing companions, to her own badness, until at last the core of her worry, namely, the image of her "bad father," could be reached.

Finally, real *analytic interpretation* was carried out on Betty's nightmares (Chapter 11) to unearth their repressed content of mourning and anxiety.

A FUTURE TECHNIQUE OF "MENTAL FIRST AID"

From the experiences collected in this book, we can perhaps extract some hints permitting us to envisage a future organized technique of "mental first aid" in the hospital, its prerequisites, its scope, its nature, and its limitations.

In view of the wide divergence in the case material and the physical afflictions of the children, such a technique will have to be flexible, i.e, applicable to disturbances which range from the surface to the depth. Since therapy is carried out within the hospital setting, it has to involve not only the parents of the patient, as in child guidance work, but equally the nursing and medical staffs. Since the approach ranges from the human to the scientific and covers every aspect of the child's life, such as physical health, illness, normal and abnormal mental life, an orientation in these various fields will be essential for the worker; so will observational skill and a thorough grounding in the essentials of a developmental child psychology.

There will always be children who can cope with traumatic happenings without therapeutic help, such as Dave (Chapter 11), as well as those whose disturbance is too severe to be influenced by a first aid scheme, such as Stephen (Chapter 12). Also beyond the scope of such a scheme will be those children who refuse to transfer allegiance from their parents, such as Ann and Judy (both in Chapter 13). Nevertheless, the majority of child patients in the hospital, whether acutely or chronically ill, will benefit greatly from any plan under which the needs of their minds are considered to be as important as the needs of their bodies.

List of Case Illustrations

ANN (8 years) 118-119, 151
  impact of mother-child interaction on arthritis
BETTY (10 years) 90-93, 146, 150
  denial and nightmare
  psychoanalytic interpretation
CARL (6 years) 106-111, 136, 141
  triumph of the mind over illness
CINDY (4½ years) 83-84, 150
  illness misunderstood as punishment
  guidance
CONNIE (2½ years) 74-75
  reaction to leg amputation
CRAIG (6 years) 68
  developmental spurt after immobilization ended
DANNY (8 years) 130
  adjustment to home after hospitalization
DAVE (9 years) 95-99, 144, 151
  mastery by constructive defenses, wit, and humor
DIANA (12 years) 75-76
  reaction to leg amputation
DONNA (10 years) 37, 61, 93-94, 144, 146
  positive relation to doctor
  cheerful acceptance (based on fantasy) of restrictive treatment
  pain reinforcing masochistic tendencies
  withdrawal and reversal
ELIZABETH (10½ years) 85-88, 138, 141, 150
  illness misunderstood as punishment
  guidance
ERNEST (8 years) 81-82, 150
  illness misunderstood as punishment for masturbation
  guidance

154   List of Case Illustrations

Eve (12 years) 38
  negative relation to doctor
Gene (adolescent) 66, 130-131, 144
  negative reaction to removal of cast
  negative adaptation
George (8 years) 37-38
  positive relation to doctor
Harriet (10-13 years) 51-53, 94-95, 143, 146, 148
  successful preparation at slow pace
  adaptation by regression
Henry (16 years) 62-63, 136
  acceptance of major procedures and protest against minor
    procedures unconnected with major illness
  breakdown of acceptance
Jackie (5 years) 55-56, 131, 136, 148
  preparation by reality confrontation
Jane (3 years) 53-54, 148, 149
  unsuccessful preparation of a three-year-old
  use of play therapy
Joel (5 years) 63-64
  acceptance of major procedures and protest against minor
    procedures unconnected with major illness
Joyce (5-15 years) 75, 121-122
  reaction to leg amputation of another child
  arthritic child's involvement with mother
  "mothering own body" in absence of mother
  defensive independence
Judy (8 years) 123-125, 128, 151
  impact of mother-child relationship on asthmatic child
Katie (4 years) 67-68
  verbalization affected by immobilization
Keith (5 years) 66-67, 143
  negative reaction to release from immobilization
Larry (8 years) 111-116, 136, 149
  requiring help to develop defenses and control
  "corrective emotional experience"
Leah (10 years) 70
  cardiac patient's preoccupation with heartbeat
Lily (adolescent) 65-66
  identification on basis of common lot
  negative reaction to removal of cast
Linda (8 years) 48-51, 136, 148
  successful preparation for surgery

List of Case Illustrations

MARION (7 years) 57-58, 125-126, 136, 144, 146, 149
  necessary preparation for minor events
  asthmatic attack tied to mother's presence
  educational intervention by therapist
MAY (3 years) 118-121, 149
  arthritic child's involvement with mother
  therapeutic handling of food refusal
  play therapy
MRS. M. 123
  influence of relationship to own mother on handling of child
NANCY (13 years) 131-132
  mother's role in guiding child's home adjustment
ROBERT (14 years) 73-74, 76, 130
  reaction of other children to blindness of
  positive adaptation
RONNIE (2½ years) 33-34, 149
  permissive nursing of very young
  "corrective emotional experience"
RUBY (4 years) 54-55, 146, 148
  despair not lessened by preparation
RUTH (9 years) 82-83, 138, 150
  illness misunderstood as punishment (for masturbation)
  guidance
SALLY (9 years) 126
  asthma not cured by dust-free atmosphere
  impact of emotional state on asthma
SAMMY (11 years) 77-78
  reaction of other children to death of
SHIRLEY (5 years) 24-25
  compliance with medical procedures after mother's
  acceptance of them
SOPHIA (13 years) 93
  denial by fantasy
STEPHEN (6 years) 101-105, 141, 143, 151
  physical illness as a destructive influence on personality
SYLVIA (adolescent) 65-66
  identification based on common lot
  negative reaction to removal of cast

Index

Adaptation
  constructive, 95-99, 151
  dependent on home atmosphere, 131-132
  to home, after hospitalization, 130-132
  not determined by degree of physical impairment, 130-131
  by regression, 94-95
Adenoidectomy, 43, 136
Admission procedures, 26-30, 129
Affect, reality of child's, 137
Aggression, 101-105
  turned against self, 105
  see also Anxiety attacks, Rebelliousness, Temper tantrums
Alleviation, see Comforting
Ambivalence, 124, 130
Amputation, 47, 137
  of leg, 54-55, 74-76
Anxiety, 12
  and asthma, 127
  break-through during recovery, 65-66
  defenses against, 29, 89-95
  displacement of, 149
  freely expressed, 28
  of parents, 13, 23
  and reality appraisal, 39
  revealed by story, 120-121
  revival of earlier, 28
  spreading through ward, 72-73
  and submission, 105
  and surgery, 44-46, 115
  and time experience, 139-140
  uncovering of, 92-93, 150
  unrealistic, 60
  see also Castration anxiety, Fantasy, Fear, Nightmare
Anxiety attacks, 105, 115
Arthritis, rheumatoid, 17-18, 117-122
Asthma, 18, 57, 122-128
  attack tied to mother's presence, 125-126
  emotional factors in, 127-128, 141
  improvement with child's separation from mother, 124-128
  not cured by dust-free surroundings, 126

Bergmann, T., 64
Blindness, reactions to, 73-74, 76, 130
Blood sample, taking of, 57-58, 144
Body
  concentration on, 29
  fears for intactness, see Anxiety, Castration anxiety, Fantasy, Fear
  mothering own, 122
Body-mind interaction, 35, 100, 141-145
  close, in very young children, 141
  factors influencing, 127
  "mind over matter," 111, 141

INDEX

Cardiac patient, *see* Heart disease
Castration, blindness symbol of, 73
Castration anxiety and fears, 44, 51-53, 144
    real vs. fantasied, 106
    see also Anxiety, Fantasy, Fear
Casts, 18-19, 47, 53-56, 93, 112, 131, 132
    experienced as protection, 56, 65-66
    negative reaction to removal of, 66
    reactions to removal of, 64-67
Child
    adaptability of, 30
    age of, and body-mind interaction, 141
    arthritic, involvement with mother, 117-122
    asthmatic, involvement with mother, 122-128
    cannot be prepared for death, 78-79
    capable of transferring allegiance from parent to nurse, 33-34, 148
    compliance with medical procedures after mother's acceptance of them, 24-25
    dependence on parents, 20, 22
    deprived of family care and health, 111-116, 149-150
    emotional vs. physical needs, 20, 141-145
    establishing contact with, 12, 113, 119, 147-148
    freely expressing despair, 28
    incapable of transferring allegiance from parents, 118-119, 151
    institutionalized, 111-116
    limited knowledge of reality, 44
    loss of friend, 92
    maintenance of family ties in hospital, 22-25
    meaning of "being nursed," 142-143
    mothering own body in absence of mother, 122
    neglected, 94, 148
    neurotic and physically ill, 105-106
    normal, 30, 31, 105-106, 147
    obedient, *see* Compliance, Submission
    obstructive behavior a result of: developmental conflicts, 14; previous experience, 14
    overcoming upsetting experience, 30
    "perfect," 28-29
    preparation by other child, 131-132
    protective attitude to other, 75-76
    reaction of seeing to blind, 73-74
    submissive, *see* Compliance, Submission
    unattached, 112-115
    week-end home visits, 23, 126
Child analysis, 13, 147
Child guidance, *see* Guidance
Child rearing, 147
Child therapy, 12
Childhood neurosis, 106
Chorea, 81
Circumcision, 144
Clarification, 106, 114; *see also* Reality confrontation
Clock, symbol of heart, 70
Clubfoot, 67
Comforting, 12, 54-55, 146, 148
Compliance, 24-25, 62-64, 107, 125, 140, 143
Congenital deformation, 53
Convalescence, 17-19
    prolonged, 60-68
    see also Recovery
"Corrective emotional experience," 113-116, 149-150
Cure, magic hope for, 62
Curiosity, 60

Deafness, 73, 130

Death, 105-106
  accidental or suicide, 105
  fear of, 92, 102-106
  impact of, 76-79
  no preparation for, 78-79
  preoccupation with, 102-106
Defenses, 89-99, 148-149
  breakdown of, 29
  noninterference with, 93-94
  uncovering of, 90-93
  see also Denial, Displacement, Regression, Repression, Reversal
Denial, 29, 70, 105
  by fantasy, 93
  by nightmare, 90-93
  primitive, 89-90
  respect for, 94, 146
Dependence, 14, 37
  enjoyment of, 94-95
  masochistic, 37; see also Masochistic tendencies
  see also Child, Passivity
Depression, 29, 118
Development
  emotional, 20-21
  oral phase, 144
  progress after removal of motor restraint, 67-68
  psychoanalytic theory of, 9, 11, 147, 151
  see also Personality development
Diets, 144
Diplegia, spastic, 48
Displacement, 70, 149
Doctor, 13-14, 18, 36
  child's relation to, 14, 20, 37-39, 45, 50, 53, 55-56, 98, 132, 135
  evaluation of illness different from child's 135-137
  object of identification, 36
  see also Medical staff
Dream, see Nightmare

Eating difficulties, 23-24, 29, 33-34, 141
  handling of, 119-120
Education, 149

Events
  meaning of, 45
  see also Illness, Medical procedures, Surgery
Explanation, see Clarification, Reality confrontation

Fantasy
  of annihilation (mutilation), 144
  anxious, 57, 148
  archaic, 127
  aroused by lack of understanding, 69
  of being attacked, 136, 144
  coincidence with reality in ill child, 106
  defense against, 29
  denial by, 93
  endurance of hardship will bring health, 61-62
  illness as confirmation of reality of, 138
  and masturbation, 81-83
  preoccupation with, 29
  spreading through ward, 72-73
  and surgery, 44-46
  see also Anxiety, Castration anxiety, Fear
Father, influence of, on child, 107-111
Fears
  absence of, in mother's presence, 118
  annihilation, 106
  archaic, 44
  fantastic, 144, 148
  and lack of reality understanding, 69
  of mutilation, 37, 136
  real vs. fantasied, 106
  of retribution, 105-106, 138
  spreading through ward, 72-73
  of wetting, 108
  see also Anxiety, Castration anxiety, Fantasy
Food
  fads, 23

INDEX 159

Food (cont'd)
  refusal, 119-120
  see also Eating difficulties
Freud, A., 45
Frustration tolerance, 44

Group, significant social, 72-73
Group situation
  help from, 60, 69
  not helped by, 69
Guidance, 12, 85-88, 104, 150-151
Guillain-Barré syndrome, 17, 37, 83
Guilt, 49, 61, 101, 138, 148, 150
  about having caused illness, 36
  over masturbation, 81-83
  over "secret," 85-88

Heart disease, 17-18, 38, 82
  emotional factors in, 141
  lack of observable factors, 69-70
  typical reactions, 68-71
Heartbeat, concentration on, 69-70
Helplessness
  of child, *see* Dependence, Submission
  of mother, 118
Hernia repair, 43, 136
Home, return to, 110-111, 116, 129-132
Hospital
  admission procedures, *see* Admission procedures
  compared to home life, 20-24, 72, 129-130
  life, meaning of, 20-21
  setting, 17-39
  source of intimate knowledge of child, 140
  visiting rules, 22-25, 72
  ward, child's social group, 72
Hospital therapist
  acting as "auxiliary ego," 148-149
  establishing contact with, 12, 113, 119, 147-148
  relation to medical staff, 13-14, 145, 151

  relation to nurses, 24-25, 32-33, 145, 151
  relation to parents, 13, 24-25, 104-105, 109
  techniques used, *see* Mental first aid
  use of information, 13-14
Hospitalization
  prolonged, 72, 111-117
  reactions to, 26-30, 124
  repeated, 18, 38, 57, 83, 90, 109, 119, 123
Humor, 95-99
Hypochondriacal attitude, 68, 122

Identification
  on basis of common lot, 60, 65-66, 69
  with other child, 76
  with staff, 20, 36
Illness
  conceived as imprisonment, 96, 110
  course of, influenced by mother, 117-128
  duration, child's conception, 138-140
  influence of emotional factors, 117-128, 141
  influence on personality development, *see* Personality development
  major impairment tolerated better than minor, 131
  mastery of, 95-99
  and masturbation, *see* Masturbation
  means of clinging to infantile relationship to mother, 124-125
  misunderstood as punishment, 80-88, 101, 110, 137-138, 144
  reactions to acute vs. chronic, 135-140
  severe vs. minor, 135-140
  typical reactions to specific, 59-71
Immobilization, 12, 24, 45, 47, 54
  reactions to, 59-67

160 INDEX

Independence, defensive, 122
Infection, 106, 137, 144
  fear of, 82, 84
Intelligence, high, and poor school performance, 102-105
Interpretation, analytic, 106, 150

Learning inhibition, 29, 102-105
Legg-Perthes disease, 17, 19, 24, 63
Loyalty conflicts, 32, 85-87, 148

Masochistic tendencies aroused by painful experience, 37, 61, 144, 149
Masturbation, 65, 86
  illness conceived as result of, 81-83, 144
Medical procedures, 12, 25, 28
  absence of fear of, in mother's presence, 118
  acceptance of, based on fantasy, 61
  breakdown of acceptance, 62-64
  child's compliance with, after mother's acceptance of, 24-25
  child's conception of, 136-137, 143-144
  evaluated differently by child and adult, 136-137
  painful, 37, 61, 142, 144
  preparation for, *see* Preparation
  protest against, 24-25; *see also* Rebelliousness
  visibility of apparatus, 60
  see also Compliance, Nursing, Submission
Medical staff
  considering emotional implications of physical needs, 142-145
  see also Doctor
Menstruation, 86
Mental first aid, 12-14
  limitations of, 14, 151
  technique, 145-151
  see also Clarification, Comforting, "Corrective emotional experience," Guidance, Hospital therapist, Play therapy, Preparation, Reality confrontation, Reassurance
Mind-body interaction, *see* Body-mind interaction
Mother
  anxiety in, 127
  child's involvement with, 24-25, 117-118
  guidance, 46-47
  guilt of, 118, 123
  helplessness of, 118
  and hospital therapist, *see* Hospital therapist
  rebellion against medical procedures used on child, 24-25
  regards child's illness as retribution for suffering inflicted on her own mother, 123
  relation to doctor, 36
  relation to nurse, *see* Nurse
  role in guiding child's adjustment, 131-132
  see also Parents
Mother-child relationship, distortions of, 122-128
Motor functions, recovery, 59-68
Motor restraint, reactions to, 29, 64-68, 138
  see also Immobilization
Mucus, swallowing of, 125
Muscle transplant, 51-53
Muscular dystrophy, 17, 77-78

Nightmares, and denial, 90-93, 150
Nurse, 13-14, 20, 24, 28, 45, 105, 122, 132
  and admission procedures, 27-28
  attachment to, 114-116
  child's relation to, 31-34, 51, 97-98, 114-116, 144
  considering emotional implications of physical care, 142-145
  relation to mothers, 24-25
  revolt against, 113
  understanding of illness different from child's, 135-137

INDEX

Nursing
  difficulties, 112-113
  meaning of, to older child, 142-143
  permissive, 33-34, 149-150
  reactions to, *see* Compliance, Medical procedures, Rebelliousness, Submissiveness
  of very young, 32-34

Oedipus complex, 37
Orthopedic cases, 18, 140
  typical reactions, 59-68

Pain, 117-122, 139
  upsets pleasure-unpleasure balance, 142
  see also Masochistic tendencies
Paraplegia, 62, 75
Parents
  anxiety of, 13, 23
  assuming responsibility for aftercare, 131
  fear of assuming responsibility for care of child, 23
  guidance of, 151
  relation to hospital staff, 112, 148
  see also Father, Hospital therapist, Mother
Passivity
  difficulty in abandoning, 66-67, 94-95
  fight against, 143
Personality development
  illness a destructive influence on, 101-105
  impact of illness on, 100-116, 130, 141-145, 147
  requirements, 20
  triumph of mind over illness, 106-111
  see also Development
Play, anticipatory, 47, 53-54
Play therapy, 119-120, 149
Poliomyelitis, 17, 33, 51, 66, 90, 94, 95, 99, 101-102, 106-111, 140

Preparation, 115, 146, 149
  and age of child, 46-48
  despair not lessened by, 54-55
  emergency, 115
  for minor events, 57-58
  by other child, 131-132
  by reality confrontation, 55-56
  at slow pace, 51-53, 146
  successful, 48-53
  unsuccessful, 53-54
Psychosomatic disorders, 127-128, 141
Punishment
  illness misunderstood as, 80-88, 101, 110, 137-138, 144
  surgery perceived as, 44

Rainbow Hospital
  admission procedures, 26-30, 129
  a long-stay hospital, 19-21, 140
  medical staff, 35
  the setting, 17-18
  visiting rules, 22-25
  see also Hospital
Reality
  coincidence of internal and external, 137
  discrepancies of inner and outer, 136
  inner and outer, 44-46, 136-137
  lack of knowledge of, 68-71
  see also Fantasy
Reality confrontation, 55-56; *see also* Clarification
Reassurance, 12, 44, 60, 140, 146
Rebelliousness, 24-25, 64-65, 122, 140, 143
Recovery
  disappointments during, 64-65
  revolt during, 64-65
Regression, 29, 33-34, 66, 95, 143
  adaptation by, 94-95
  of previously achieved controls and functions, 33-34, 67-68
Repression, 92, 150
Respirator, 92, 96, 107-109, 136

Reversal
of affect, 93-94
constructive, 95-99
Rheumatic fever, 81-82, 85, 137

Sarcoidosis, 73
School
avoidance, 108
expulsion from, 104
in hospital, 19
inhibition of performance in, 102-105
Scoliosis, 56, 110
Separation
anxiety, 27
beneficial effect, 128
from home, 30, 140
from mother, 33-34, 48, 118
Sex organs, anomaly of, 52
Sleep difficulties, 29, 141
Soiling, 29, 33-34
Spina bifida, 66-67
Stealing, 113-115
Stomach upsets, 138, 141
Submission, 29-30, 93-94, 101, 105, 107, 125
Surgery
acceptance of, and rebellion against minor, 62-64
child's conceptions of, 136-137
conceived as castration, 51-53
corrective, 17, 19, 44, 105
postoperative phase, 47, 54, 56
preparation for, 43-58; *see also* Preparation
repeated, 18, 27-28, 98
spinal, 55-56, 65, 93, 99

Symptoms, transitory neurotic, 108

Temper tantrums, 29, 62 68, 102, 113, 115
Time, child's conception of, 138-140
Toddler
difficulties in preparation for surgery, 47-48
need for mother, 32-34, 48
nursing of, 32-34
and postponement of wish fulfillment, 139
see also Child, Development, Personality development
Toilet training, 33, 124-125
Tonsillectomy, 43, 136
Tooth extraction, 62, 82
Toy, special, 53-54, 63, 70
Traction, 47, 54, 66, 112
Tuberculosis, 19, 140
of bones and joints, 17, 111
of spine, 37, 93

Veeneklaas, N. G. M., 146
Verbalization, regression in, 67-68
Visiting, 112, 117, 120, 126; *see also* Hospital

Weaning, 124-125
Wetting, 29, 33-34
Wish fulfillment, postponement of, 139
Wit, 95-99
Withdrawal, emotional, 29-30, 71, 93-94, 101, 107, 118-119, 140